THE COLD WAR

Arm Yourself Against
Colds & Viruses

THE COLD WAR

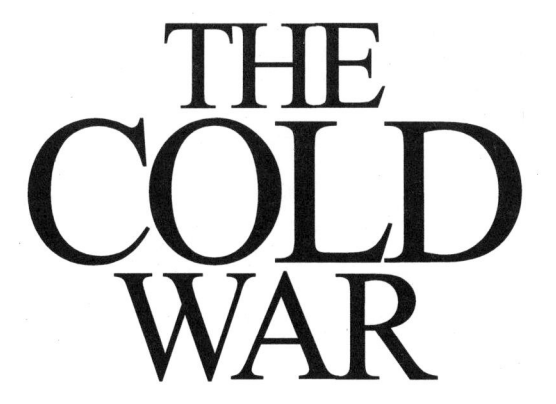

Arm Yourself Against Colds & Viruses

Malcolm Newell MA, PhD

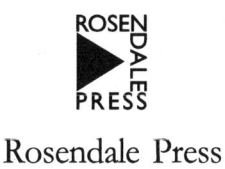

Rosendale Press

Copyright © 1996 Malcolm Newell

First published in Great Britain in 1996 by
Rosendale Press Ltd
Premier House
10 Greycoat Place
London SW1P 1SB

First published in Australia in 1995 by
Stirling Press Ltd

All rights reserved. No part of this publication may be reproduced, stored in a retrieval system, or transmitted, in any form or by any means, electronic, mechanical, photocopying, recording or otherwise, without the prior permission of the copyright owners.

The right of Malcolm Newell as author of this work has been asserted by him in accordance with the Copyright, Designs and Patents Act, 1993.

Jacket design by Pep Reiff
Printed in the United Kingdom by the Cromwell Press

British Library Cataloguing in Publication Data
A catalogue record for this book is available from The British Library

ISBN 1 872803 36 9

Contents

Introduction 7

1 Causes of the common cold 13
At least 200 viruses • Why you can't resist them all • Situations that make you vulnerable • Health versus sickness • Catching cold • Symptoms and signs • How a cold differs from the flu or a bacterial infection • The course of a cold • What a cold tells you • When a cold is something else

2 Research since World War II 27
From cold feet to megadoses of vitamins • The cold 'farm' in Britain • Getting paid to have a cold • Bolting the stable door…treating symptoms not causes • Viruses, not bacteria • Byways and quirks of common cold viruses • Blind alleys

3 Tablets and other treatments 39
'Go to bed with a hot lemon and honey…' • The aspirin/paracetamol approach • The ubiquitous antibiotic • Sore throats and swollen glands • Preventing a more serious outcome • Age and resistance • Flu injections and misconceptions • A mine of misinformation

4 How the immune system works 51
The basis and process of immunity • Vitamins are only bit players in the orchestra • Sunshine and susceptibility • Structures of general health • Getting 'run down' • Reversing the downward slide to disease • Why viruses evolve and mutate • Individual quirks and complications • How immunity is built

5 More pieces of the puzzle   61
Who gets sick and why? • The synthesis of mind and body • Red herrings: How diet vitamins can help • An orange a day keeps... • Why the story is much more complex • 'Health' foods and foolish fads • Genetic antecedents

6 How diet, sunshine and activity interact   77
The chemistry of sunlight • Vitamin D synthesis • Promoting the wonders of sunlight • Tanning and the fear of cancers • The effects of sun deprivation • The role of light for a living photo-cell • How the pineal gland plays a part • Summer and winter ills • Where exercise plays a vital role • The energy/output balance • Fresh and wholesome – the crime of the cook

7 Effects of an industrial lifestyle   91
Why do some succumb – but not others? • Workload and stresses • That air conditioning system... • The mismanagement of heating • Urban life and resistance • Lifestyle and other aggravations • Pollutants and air quality • The factors we need not consider

8 Never have another cold   99
The culture of the common cold • Building effective resistance • Physical fitness – for life • Prevention is better than cure • Assessing the immune system's health • Picking the first indications • What to do if you still start to succumb • Suppressing the symptoms for 48 hours • The minefield of the mind

Conclusion   113

Index   121

Introduction

Have you ever wondered why some people never get colds? Just luck? Or some fortunate genetic inheritance that has bequeathed on them sparkling good health? In a kinder moment you could even put their good health down to better lifestyle management. In the meantime, you pack up your paper tissues to head off for another day of snuffles and embarrassment at work.

Research scientists have been studying the common cold intensely since World War II. At one research institution, volunteers were actually paid to have cold viruses injected into them to induce a cold. But apart from identifying at least 200 viruses that can produce cold or flu symptoms, we have not travelled far down the road to a reliable cure. Certainly, we can give those at risk flu injections, primarily for types A and B, or a locally identified form, but for those people who are not immunised the best we can do is send them to bed with lemon and honey and let them sweat it out.

Ah but, you say, my doctor – we'll call him or her a physician in this book – always gives me a prescription for an antibiotic when I turn up to the surgery with flu. He does? Well, should he? Or is that part of the problem?

Antibiotics are the wonder drug of the 20th century but they cannot cure any of the viruses that *cause* the common cold. They are anti-bacterial agents which today, because of misuse and over-prescription, are rapidly losing healing power as the bad bugs mutate and adapt to antibiotic attack. New forms of antibiotic are being developed to answer the problem of increasing bacterial resistance, and the so-called broad spectrum antibiotics are still effective for many specific complaints but, as a general cure-all to salve an uncertain physician's conscience or protect his legal indemnity premium, the days of over prescription are numbered.

An antibiotic cannot do a workmanlike job when you are seriously ill, or when a life threatening condition like pneumonia threatens, if your immunity has been compromised by excessive use, particularly in childhood. If every wheeze or sniffle identified by a fussy mother is so treated, a child matures without arming the powerful defence systems of the body and so is at much greater risk later.

The key to health is the body's complex immune system.

An illness is not the result of attack by an external agent – *it is a failure of the body's immune system.* That is a basic and vital concept to grasp first. As long as we choose to avoid any responsibility by blaming an agent outside ourselves, we cannot marshal the necessary forces of good health.

Raising a child is more than nurturing and providing medical care and education. A parent also has a duty to develop the child's physical resources and capabilities through adequate diet, exercise, sensible exposure to sunlight and clean air, and the effective management of childhood ills. The sequence of relatively minor ailments confers on susceptible children a lifelong immunity to many common diseases and minor infections, or at least an enhanced and effective system of defences against bacterial, viral or fungal attack.

In the industrialised and urbanised world of today, many aspects of our relatively comfortable lifestyles – for most people but not all – provide ideal conditions for the transmission and incubation of cross infections. Let's get one point straight now. Most of the bugs that cause the symptoms we variously label 'a cold' or 'the flu' are ever-present in any community and, probably, any body. Something happens at some point to predispose that body's defences to surrender to one of the waiting attackers.

To rid oneself of the threat of repeated and debilitating colds, it is necessary to find out why you are succumbing to these infections and so maintain health and immunity that any new exposure to infection cannot conclude in illness. That does not mean, however, that you will be immune to every form of viral or bacteriological attack. The body's repertoire of immunity, of being able to recognise and deal with pathogens, increases in much the same way that a musician learns new works.

As we mature through childhood, there are two main sources of developing immunity – that acquired either genetically or from our mothers at birth or during breast feeding and, secondly, by exposure to a myriad of infections that produce troublesome but relatively minor and unthreatening symptoms.

Left alone without drug interference, most children will bounce back quickly and be armed against that particular pathogen when next they encounter it. A child in good health – there lies the key – will resist many common infections and develop immunity rapidly and effectively for those he or she has not otherwise been equipped to counter.

A good example of this is susceptibility to malaria, one of the world's most extensive and troublesome diseases in hot countries. A visitor to the tropics, once bitten by an infected mosquito, may succumb quickly because the body's defences do not recognise this new threat and have no means of dealing with it. A local may also succumb to the disease, perhaps because of reduced immunity resulting from poor diet or arduous living conditions, but the effect and severity of the disease will be much less than the impact on the visiting stranger.

If we were not fortunate enough to maximise immunity in childhood, all is not lost. Once you understand the function of the immune system – and how mind and body interact and function in accord with the broader physical environment, the possibility of dramatically increasing the range and power of the immune system can be realised. Beating the common cold, and no longer falling prey to every passing pathogen, does not call for any arduous health regime, just some simple commonsense measures and, perhaps, a few changes of attitude.

In this book, we're going to move far beyond the rather crude proposition that became popular in the 1970s, mainly as a consequence of some 'ground breaking' work on the interactions of vitamin C and the white cells that form part of the immune system. Media reports of this research prompted many people to rush out and buy high dose ascorbic acid tablets dressed up in fizziness to ward off colds and other infections. Most were probably rather surprised when the ploy failed miserably, though, had they been injured or broken a bone, they may have shortened the recovery time if they were prepared to put up with the resulting intestinal inconvenience.

Still, it was good business for drug manufacturers and pharmacies and who's to argue with people pumping a bit more vitamin C into deficient diets in our supermarket culture of overcooking and freezing. If you ingested too much, the body simply excreted the surplus so megadoses of up to three grams a day, it was argued, couldn't do much harm. Well, we now know such dosage levels could exacerbate gastric ulcers or heighten acidity because the causal bacterium, *Helicobacter pylori*, thrives in an acidic environment.

There were other problems. What we were doing, in simple analogy, was tuning up one instrument in an orchestra that was playing out of tune.

In *The Cold War*, we're going to show how you can tune up the whole orchestra to a point where the resulting music – a healthy and resistant mind and body – is harmonious and the basis of a long and disease-free life, as far as is practically possible. Along the way, we're going to discard many of the myths of 'catching cold' or when to seek medical help. The focus will shift towards taking personal responsibility for your health and not sloughing it off onto an overworked physician who hasn't got the time to delve into the byways of your physical shortcomings, however much he or she may wish so to do.

Even with a relatively minor change of view, any reader of this book should be able to reduce, if not eliminate, the common cold as an ever present threat to daily life, particularly in the gloomy depths of winter. After all, the common cold is more than a part of Anglo-Saxon folklore, it's an element of our culture! In childhood we learn we will inevitably 'catch cold' and suffer the resulting unpleasantness.

Since developing and refining the research on the common cold that underlies this book, and applying the simple principles involved, I've succumbed to one viral infection, probably a strain of flu following overseas travel (1986) to which I had no developed antibodies, and one minor throat ailment, probably a streptococcal infection (1989). In both cases, there were compelling reasons why my immunity was compromised at that time. A simple readjustment of lifestyle has prevented any further 'mistakes'. If I had known at the outset what I know now, both these illnesses could have been avoided easily enough.

(Just in case you make similar 'mistakes' in the early days, the final chapter will offer a failsafe technique to suppress the symptoms and prevent the worst effects from developing at all.)

Enough of personal experience. Without firm conviction, I couldn't have written this book. The hard evidence, backed up by argument and observation, will speak for itself. Then you can experiment yourself, apply the prescriptions, and discover that the approach outlined here *really does work*.

To convince yourself of this, however, you need to negotiate the preliminary steps and understand the causes of the common cold, or flu, the course it takes, and why you succumb when others do not. Unless you are convinced that the propositions set down are correct and effective, you will not be able to engineer the level of immunity needed to ward off the more troublesome bugs that have a go at you from day to day.

We'll consider the present conventional wisdom and medical outlook and set these views in the context of the pressures which prompt physicians to act as they do in trying circumstances, legal and organisational. Much of the trite 'advice' pumped out by popular magazines and alleged 'health' experts will be subjected to critical appraisal because, unless we sort out the real issues, we can't get the immune system functioning properly.

Along the way we'll discover that some of the most favoured treatments to alleviate cold and flu symptoms really make things worse. They are truly 'good for a cold' because they prolong the cycle of infection – and the discomfort and disablement that goes with it. And we'll consider some other popular propaganda foisted on an unsuspecting public in the name of government that promises not only to make them progressively less resistant to disease but, more alarmingly, affect the well-being of their children for life.

This is not an eccentric view.

There is a battery of intelligent and well qualified medical and scientific opinion sitting unread in every library in the land to support this argument. It's all there for anyone to digest if they really want to end the scourge of the common cold.

Next time you succumb to that unpleasant and intrusive infection, curl up in a warm bed with a lemon and honey (at least *that* won't do you any harm), and take this medicine a chapter at a time until you reach a point where you resolve to stay healthy instead.

CHAPTER 1

CAUSES OF THE COMMON COLD

According to the May 1995 issue of *Current Therapeutic Research*, infections of the upper respiratory tract – those we generally label a cold or flu – are among the most common complaints encountered in medical practice or hospitals. Most of these infections are sinusitis, acute bacterial forms of chronic bronchitis, pharyngitis and pneumonia. Of these illnesses, streptococci bacteria cause about a third. Some nine different micro-organisms are responsible for nearly all cases of community acquired respiratory tract infection. The other two thirds are caused by viral agents. Of these, hundreds have been identified so far – and there are more to find.

In bacteriological terms, it's a big bad world out there. But anyone who takes the view that catching a cold is a lottery in which, magically, one avoids infection by chance and good luck should think again. At any one moment, there is a vast array of pathogens ready to fulfil their lifecycle dictates by attacking a human host.

This is precisely why a view of illness that relies on blaming an agent outside oneself for any breakdown in health is inadequate. There is more to the story than cause and effect.

In the most recent edition of the *Cecil Textbook of Medicine*, the authors point out that many viral infections have characteristics that make clear diagnosis possible – those that cause, for example, measles, mumps, chicken pox and polio. But many other viruses do not produce clearly definable symptoms. In fact, 200 or more distinct viruses may cause the common cold and related disorders.

These can be sub-divided into roughly 100 types of rhinoviruses which produce 15-40 per cent of common colds, and coronaviruses, which produce 10-20 per cent of colds. Add to these the flu viruses which cause so much winter misery – influenza A, B, C and mutations – four types of parainfluenza virus, respiratory syncytial virus and adenoviruses of several types, and you account for another five to 10 per cent of colds. Last on this daunting list is the Coxsachie virus and some echoviruses which cause up to two per cent of colds. And the streptococci bacterium referred to above is thought to produce symptoms identified as 'a cold' in two to 10 per cent of cases.

Apart from these pathogens, there is no readily identifiable agent responsible though all other colds (30-50 per cent) are thought to be caused by an unidentified virus.

The common cold is the most frequently occurring ailment in humans worldwide. In 1981 in the United States, it was estimated that 93 million colds were endured by sufferers. That runs out to more than 40 colds per 100 people a year and roughly one fifth of all the acute conditions treated by physicians. This represents a massive cost to the community in lost working time and delivering medical services and drugs.

In the Cleveland Family Study spanning 10 years and including a review of more than 25,000 illnesses, the common cold represented 60 per cent of all sickness. Included under the heading of the common cold in this study, were rhinitis, laryngitis, bronchitis and other acute upper respiratory infections. The astounding conclusion was that sufferers across all age groups *averaged* almost six infections a year. This suggests that some people were getting more than six colds a year. Children under one averaged seven colds a year, rising to more than eight during the second year of life, and remaining at this high level until age five when they were still getting an average of more than seven colds a year. From age six, when most children are at school, the incidence fell to around four colds a year, the adult rate. Boys were shown to be more vulnerable than girls but, in adults, mothers were more vulnerable than fathers. The rate of infection was higher in schoolgoers than in children kept at home. And the number of colds increased as family size increased, a curious finding which raises questions about the development of immunity.

The study claims that roughly one quarter of all exposures to viruses in the home result in an illness. How we know this is questionable, of course. A more recent American study in Michigan estimated a mean three colds per person year with one year olds succumbing to six or more infections, and one to two year olds slightly fewer than six. Rhinoviruses were thought to account for 40 per cent of these illnesses.

Worldwide, human antibodies to rhinoviruses are found in industrial countries, throughout the Third World and even in tropical regions. This immunity, you'll be pleased to discover, continues to build into adult life. In temperate climates, colds occur primarily in the cold months with a general pattern of low summer incidence and high winter rates of infection. The winter rate in the United States, for example, is roughly double that of summer. In the northern hemisphere, isolating the months November to March, the coldest months, lifts the average number of colds per person to seven a year.

A similar pattern exists in the southern hemisphere though, as will be argued later, there are geographical and lifestyle factors to account for marked differences in some regions and peoples.

In the *Cecil Textbook of Medicine* (1988), the focus is on infetion based on contact, an exposure to pathogens as the basis for acquiring colds – the 'external agent' view. To demonstrate this point, some researchers in 15 trials recovered viruses from fingers that had touched plastic surfaces contaminated by rhinoviruses one to three hours earlier. They found the virus could be transmitted directly from hand to hand by touching in 11 of 15 cases, while exposure to particles from coughing and sneezing was a much less efficient mode of transmission – only the bigger particles presented a route of transmission. Married and childless couples without rhinovirus immunity transmitted the virus from one to the other in 38 per cent of the cases tested, even though it was discovered that the presence of the virus in saliva was 'not strongly associated with transmission'.

In what is known as the Spitzbergen Study, exposure to cold in whatever form, what our grandparents used to call a 'chill', was found to have no significant effect either on resistance, that is immunity, or inducing cold symptoms – symptoms indicating the common cold. In this region, fewer colds occurred during the bitter Arctic weather but there were sudden sharp outbreaks after the arrival of a ship as the weather warmed.

Was this a result of exposure to new causal agents or lowered immunity at the end of winter?

These studies showed that the essential trigger was exposure to infected individuals. Even fatigue and sleep deprivation does not seem to affect the rate of infection though, in women, susceptibility to colds was related to the menstrual cycle. That is, *attempts to induce colds during menstruation were relatively unsuccessful.*

The incubation period of a cold is three to five days but most viral infections develop in about two days.

Virus shedding, that is the ability of the infected person to pass on the virus, starts with the onset of the symptoms and continues for about a week or slightly longer. All 100 types of rhinovirus circulate in the community simultaneously for most of the year, but there are peaks in autumn and spring. In the northern hemisphere, for example, these viruses are least prevalent in the coldest months, December, January and February, even though colds still occur. The causal agent in the coldest months may not be a rhinovirus but the coronavirus which has a different lifecycle.

Some viruses have a two to four year cycle of activity which differs from place to place. Though reinfection can occur, most of these viruses once encountered produce partial or lasting immunity. That is, the body's defences, a healthy immune system, can identify and deal with the villain when it attacks.

In the case of the rhinovirus, the major symptom in 50-60 per cent of cases is nasal congestion, rhinorrhea (runny nose), and sneezing. Half of those infected will have a sore throat, and one quarter or more will be hoarse and develop a persistent cough. A high temperature is unusual, however, occurring in less than one per cent of sufferers. About a quarter of those infected will report headaches. The illness lasts from four to nine days, with most people aware of the symptoms for about a week. Rhinoviruses are not significant contributors to bronchitis, pneumonia or croup in children but they are implicated in asthma attacks in known sufferers.

Symptoms produced by the coronavirus are similar to the rhinovirus but there are also muscular and general aches, alternating shivering and fever, and nasal congestion. The virus takes slightly longer to incubate, about a day more, but is shorter in duration though there is more nasal discharge during this time.

Complications include sinusitis, and extensions of infections to the central nervous and cardiovascular systems. A viral infection may also develop alongside, or prompt, a bacterial infection leading to much more serious complications – the key reason why physicians resort to wide use of antibiotics to prevent the development of complications following a viral infection. There's another problem. Rhinovirus and coronavirus infections can mimic infections caused by bacterial streptococci which can be treated effectively with antibiotics, though this should be avoided unless there are indications of more serious complications.

Removal of the tonsils in children does not, the *Cecil Textbook* asserts, appear to affect the rate of common cold occurrence and big doses of vitamin C do not reduce the rate of infection though there is evidence that they may mitigate the course of the illness. However, a deficiency of the vitamin can increase vulnerability.

So what chance of producing a rhinovirus vaccine?

This is probably impossible because of the number of discrete infectious agents under this heading. One would have to develop the vaccine for each of the different viruses as it is unlikely that any form of general protection could ever be developed. The boosting of immunity, however, with interferon or the like given in nasal sprays can reduce the number of infections but this is useless once the symptoms have appeared. There have even been attempts to develop viricidal tissues. The conclusions reached later in this book remove the need for that kind of approach.

Interferon as a means of boosting the immune system is at best a last resort after other and more natural methods fail. Interferon used as a protective can reduce the severity and duration of the infection of colds induced by coronaviruses but it is not practical for general use because it is difficult to manufacture and very costly.

While considering the infection normally labelled a 'cold', there should be some focus on similar conditions, all of which tend to get lumped into one category – colds or flu. These include viral pharyngitis, laryngitis, croup and bronchitis, all infections that strike at the upper and middle respiratory passages and produce acute inflammation with the severity of the response depending on the site.

Keep in mind here that inflammation reveals the protective work of the immune system.

Croup occurs only in children, usually in the second year of life. It begins abruptly and abates after five to 10 days. The viral agents responsible can include rhinovirus, coronavirus, influenza A or B, adenoviruses, parainfluenza, enteroviruses and respiratory syncytial viruses. This will give you some idea of the problem facing your physician when you or one of your children presents cold symptoms, or croup. There's little chance of identifying the causal agent without extensive testing and it doesn't really matter anyway. The physician's task is to ensure that the virus does not cause more serious damage, or more precisely, to be aware of when more serious complications are likely to occur and to act before they can do any serious damage.

So, as a general diagnostic rule, if the sufferer has a runny nose, what the physician terms coryza, the common cold is present in whatever form.

Respiratory syncytial virus (RSV) occurs each year from autumn to spring, over about five months in all, with almost half the infections caused occurring in a 'peak' month which can come early or late depending on climatic or other conditions. This is one of those 'bugs that are going round'. In epidemic periods, RSVs are one of the most common causes of hospital acquired infections in children's wards. The risk of acquiring such an infection rises sharply in hospital stays of more than one week, which suggests that the child's immature immune system is increasingly under attack or compromised by the sheer weight of the attack.

With this virus, reinfection is common – though many infections will produce a level of temporary immunity and develop a more long term resistance to severe lower respiratory tract conditions.

This brings us inevitably to 'the flu'. At some periods in history, influenza viruses have raged through urban communities causing high levels of death and serious complications. Epidemics of varying severity, in part depending on the form of the virus responsible, occur almost every winter though some of the reported cases are almost certainly caused by cold viruses that produce symptoms almost indistinguishable from true flu.

The influenza A virus changes, mutates, frequently. B, and the more recently identified C virus, have not been studied as intensely though they are structurally similar. It appears that the genetic variations occur less frequently with the B virus and may not occur at all with C type viruses. Or, if they do, we haven't found one yet. What the researchers call antigenic drift – minor variations in genetic structure of the organism – occur constantly with the new forms transmitted more easily between the human hosts because the level of antibody protection in any community is much lower.

Major genetic variations seem to occur in viral agents when two or more viruses infect a single host cell simultaneously. According to Cecil: 'Such an event results (in a virus) that is completely new in comparison with the presently circulating strain. Because of the high level of immunity to the old strain and lack of immunity to the new strain within the human population, the new strain, provided that it possesses intrinsic viral properties such as virulence and transmissibility, can readily cause a major outbreak of flu.'

And it can do this, of course, before the researchers and drug manufacturers can get to grips with its character and prepare a vaccine.

Local epidemics begin suddenly, peak in two to three weeks,

and last usually for five to six weeks. Reports of child infections usually indicate the onset of a flu epidemic and this is normally followed by a rise in adult reports of infection with rising hospital admissions for pneumonia, worsening chronic obstructive pulmonary disease or even congestive heart failure. Epidemics occur almost exclusively in the winter months, perhaps when immunity is a low point for reasons we will discuss later. This means flu outbreaks are most likely to occur from May to September in the southern hemisphere and October to April in the northern climes.

In an epidemic, typically from 10-20 per cent of the population are infected, though in certain populations or age groups, this rate of infection can be as high as 40-50 per cent. In the Asian flu epidemic of the late 1960s whole families fell ill. In my own family of five, only one child – the eldest – did not succumb and it's interesting to speculate on why this might have been so.

During any epidemic, there may be a new strain in circulation alongside other more 'established' varieties so A and B viruses may be active alongside RSVs. The virulent strains circulating at the end of the epidemic of the 'flu season' are most likely to cause the following season's outbreak. This knowledge helps in the advance preparation of sufficient stocks of vaccine for people most at risk of serious complications.

Pandemics occur with the arrival of a new strain, what is in effect a new virus, to which no one has any immunity. The effect can spread worldwide in this era of air travel, though the new strain is unlikely to establish itself in the opposite hemisphere until the cold season starts.

Influenza A viruses caused pandemics in 1870, 1889, 1918 at the conclusion of World War I, 1957, 1968 and 1977. The outbreaks of 1889, 1918 and 1957 were severe while the 1977 outbreak was mild by comparison. Strains prevalent in 1957, 1968 and 1977 all appear to have originated in mainland China and spread east and west to Russia and Western Europe before reaching the American continent. (One trusts that wasn't just anti-Communist propaganda.)

After one or more pandemics, the general level of immunity in the population rises. Though the outbreak occurs in the cold season, factors that cause the epidemic to taper off sharply after five to six weeks are not understood because, at this stage, only a proportion of those susceptible have been infected. Neither is it known where the virus 'hides' between epidemics or pandemics though it would almost certainly have to have a human host who is immune to its effects.

After infection, incubation takes 18 to 72 hours. The symptoms are fever, shivering, headache, myalgia (muscle pain) and malaise. In severe cases, there is prostration (exhaustion), myalgia and headache, the severity related to the degree of fever. Arthralgia (joint pain) is common. There may also be photophobia (abnormal sensitivity to light), watery eyes, and a burning sensation or pain on moving the eyes. This can all be accompanied by a dry cough, nasal discharge, nasal obstruction, hoarseness or a dry sore throat.

The temperature rises rapidly to 38-40 degrees C, occasionally even higher, within 12 hours of the onset of the symptoms. The illness usually peaks after three days, then gradually subsides – though it can last for five days or more. At the outset, the sufferer appears flushed, with hot and moist skin, eyes watery and red, and nose streaming. As these initial symptoms decline, the respiratory signs and symptoms appear with a cough developing in three to four days. The cough and lassitude, and general malaise, may persist for one or two weeks before full recovery.

In some cases, it is difficult to distinguish between an infection caused by a flu virus and those produced by other viral agents or bacteria that can generate symptoms of headache, muscle aches, fever and cough. Other respiratory viruses can produce flu like symptoms as can the streptococcus responsible for pharyngitis. In an epidemic, however, with clear general symptoms widely evident, diagnosis is simpler.

As we have already pointed out, there is no drug that is effective against these flu viruses so the only treatment is palliative, that is to ensure that a susceptible patient is as comfortable as possible and does not develop pneumonia or other respiratory conditions that could be life threatening. In the past, a drug – amantadine –

has sometimes been prescribed to shorten the duration of the fever and other symptoms by up to half. The usual dose is 100-200 milligrams daily, taken orally for three to five days. In 1988, a new form of this drug, rimantadine, came onto the market and is said to be more effective.

Apart from that, it's aspirin or paracetamol to relieve the headache and muscle pains and bring the temperature down, backed up by cough suppressants. More about the problems with this approach later.

Flu vaccines give protection against influenza viruses A and B to about 80 per cent of users. The vaccines are updated annually to target current forms of the viruses in circulation. Some people react to the vaccines – about one to two per cent of recipients may develop fever and flu symptoms after eight to 12 hours and up to a quarter of recipients may have a mild local reaction at the site of the vaccination. But there are two forms of vaccine – 'split' and 'whole' – and the split form causes fewer reactions.

Priority for vaccination is given to people with a heart or lung condition that requires ongoing medical care. Residents of nursing homes and other chronic care facilities are high on the list, as are the aged (65 plus) who are particularly vulnerable. Likewise, physicians, and nursing and support staff in hospitals are usually given protection, particularly in a flu epidemic.

Amantadine and rimantadine seem to offer some protection against influenza A and either drug can be used to support vaccination programs. As a preventative during an epidemic, the usual dose is 100 to 200 milligrams daily, taken orally. In extreme cases, of course, there is also interferon.

Last on the list of significant viral agents is the adenovirus which can infect the respiratory system or even the eyes. This virus is thought to cause up to five per cent of all the 'clinically apparent' infections in children up to the age of 10 and is usually transmitted by person to person contact or infected swimming pool water. A form of pneumonia caused by the adenovirus usually lasts for one to two weeks. There is no effective treatment but bacterially caused complications are unusual and death is rare.

Viruses generally seem to account for up to 15 per cent of

cases of pneumonia in adults and, possibly, almost half the incidence of pneumonia in children.

To digress a moment, in the January 1995 edition of *Medical Hypotheses*, a journal that indulges in some fascinating medical speculations, it was observed that flu epidemics do not seem to appear on a random basis but just before the maximum level of sunspot activity every 11 years or so. Solar activity varies widely and the cycles can be as short as seven years and as long as 16 years. Solar flares produce massive electromagnetic pulses with radio waves ranging over a wide spectrum from long radio waves to the X-ray region of the spectrum. This produces magnetic storms and the aurora well known to navigators of ships and aircraft.

Sunspot cycles, it is suggested, may link with flu epidemics, malignant melanomas, birthrates, epileptic seizures, hip breakages in old ladies, immune function, disruptive social activity and even lifespan. This would be rather hard to research or prove, however.

This account of the complex underworld of viral agents, and their bacterial counterparts, has made it quite clear that resistance, immunity, is not a simple process. No one can resist all the viral or bacteriological assaults on their body unless they have acquired immunity from parents through their genes, or breast feeding, had vaccinations against particularly threatening pathogens to develop immunity, or endured the illness in a relatively mild form so the immune system can in future recognise the bug and deal with it accordingly.

But consider how it is that physicians, hospital staff and inveterate travellers or aircrew cope with the huge range of pathogenic assaults they encounter. You will quickly realise that the wider one's exposure to hostile agents, the more efficient the individual immune response becomes. Provided that the individual is not placed at greater risk because of poor general health, being 'run down', the immune system can handle the workload with increasing effectiveness.

This suggests, then, that the key to good health is not the level of exposure to pathogens but *the overall efficiency of the immune system.* That, however, is not as simple as it sounds either.

Certain situations make a person vulnerable to attack by viruses, bacteria or fungal agents. These same situations which undermine health and the functioning of the immune system may also predispose a person to other serious medical problems. The best known example is the bereaved spouse who develops cancer or some other serious disease after the death of a lifelong partner. Travellers returning from the opposite hemisphere and subjected to long flights also seem to be especially vulnerable. People who are stressed or overworked. Patients in hospitals recovering from other ailments or operations. Anyone who is seriously depressed or under constant negative pressure. Workers in coal mines or on night shifts deprived of adequate sunlight.

The list is long. In all these situations, the body's defences are strained or undermined and an individual is put at much greater risk. Introduce another element – poor diet, stress, travel, psychological deprivation – and that may well be the factor that determines infection.

There is, however, another and critical component. In the list above, we included people who were depressed or stressed. A key factor in illness, or rather in susceptibility to infection, is a person's state of mind. More than that, an individual can create in themselves a state of susceptibility if they *expect* to succumb to illness, or if they want for whatever reason to be sick, or if they simply fear illness and form negative assessments of the world around them. Mind and body are part of a co-ordinated organism in which each relies on the other to function adequately or efficiently and in which the hormonal and chemical balances of anyone affect, or even determine, health and behaviour.

When you succumb to a cold, it's time to ask some searching questions about yourself if you really want to be rid of constant reruns in the future.

Why did my immune system fail? Did I encounter a virus or other agent that was new to me and for which I had no immunity, or was there some other reason why my body didn't cope? Did I wish this on myself for some reason?

A cold can be seen as a warning sign that you are getting

something wrong provided you subscribe to the view that you do not have to suffer every conceivable viral/bacterial/fungal form to develop effective immunity. If, however, you are convinced that immunity is only forged in the cauldron of sickness, that removes a lot of responsibility from your shoulders. It doesn't explain, though, why some people succumb to every outbreak or epidemic but the greater majority – who may never have encountered that pathogen before – do not.

In the early years of the testing of nuclear weapons, thousands of unsuspecting people were used as guinea pigs by the authorities to research the effects of radiation. Only some of these people many years later developed diseases commonly identified as a response to over exposure to radiation, in particular thyroid cancers and leukemia. Many who were exposed to very high levels of radiation are fit and well today. I've met some of these people and can testify to that. Why did they not succumb like their associates? The nuclear accident at Chernobyl in the Ukraine provides similar examples. Tens of thousands of people were harmed, some fatally, and others will die in the future as a consequence. But many were not and we need to know why this is so.

We're drawing a long bow from the banality of the common cold though the principles involved are in essence the same. A cold may be more than just a cold, it can be a clear sign that it's time to take yourself in hand and get the immune system into top gear again, just as it was a few years ago when you were always fit and well.

One other point.

Have you noticed how you tend to become sick when you can afford to be out of action for a time – when the exams are over (or before they start if you're panic stricken and you know you going to fail), when you start your holidays (or when you go back to work after a great break), when you've just completed that arduous and compelling project or assignment overseas. We seem to have some mental control over physical responses to assaults on our immune system and it is this to which we must look for *essential clues to the process* of staying healthy.

CHAPTER 2

RESEARCH SINCE WORLD WAR II

World War II focused British interest in research on the common cold so, when the Americans went home and vacated a wartime hospital at Salisbury in southern England, the property was handed over to the British Government, which set it up as the Common Cold Research Unit. A scientist, Sir Christopher Andrewes, was placed in charge of research and he wrote an account of the unit's work in two books, *The Common Cold* (1965) and *In Pursuit of the Common Cold* (1973).

Very little was known about colds until 1965, either in Britain or elsewhere in the industrialised world. Research centred on Britain in particular, in part because the relatively warm and damp climate and relatively low light intensity created a perfect environment for cold viruses to thrive.

Andrewes notes at the outset: '... if as much money was put in common cold research as was used to put men on the moon, the problem could be solved.' We have had to wait another 50 years and still only the bare bones of a lasting anti-cold strategy are now emerging. This book, finally, brings together and synthesises the world wide research of the intervening years which shows that the common cold is beatable, an outcome which would no doubt have made Andrewes a happy man.

By the time Andrews wrote his second book, 11,000 volunteers had spent one or more stays of 10 days at Salisbury to help build some basic knowledge about how and why the cold prospered and seemed invincible.

The work started promptly in 1946. The goal was to identify the pathogen that caused colds and find a cure, or a means of preventing the disease. At this time, most viruses were thought to have been identified but, as Andrewes says, 'the common cold was one of the few infections that remained quite baffling'. All but a few diehard bacteriologists believed the cause was probably a virus.

Dr Alphonse Dochez and colleagues in New York started the hunt first in 1926 and quickly ruled out any bacterial agent as the main cause. Andrewes started his research at Saint Bartholomew's Hospital in London with a colleague, Dr W. G. Oakley, in 1931 with the help of some students who were to be the 'guinea pigs' because they were cheaper to use than the then customary chimpanzees. By 1933, Andrewes was attempting to locate the cause of influenza as well, but using ferrets this time instead of students.

The Salisbury cold unit was ideally situated in the former US Army's Harvard Hospital. The 16-acre property was relatively remote and consisted of 38 or so separate prefabricated buildings. The only other requirements apart from staff were large stocks of paper hankies. As an additional luxury, there was a huge old sofa donated by the departing Americans. The whole establishment was light and airy, sometimes rather too airy given the vigorous south-westerly gales that roared across the open land around.

Recruiting volunteers was difficult at first so Andrewes once again resorted to university students. Soon the unit was the butt of music hall jokes and a source of interest for the media. The volunteers had to be aged at least 18 and no more than 40, though the upper limit was later extended to 50 when it was discovered that the over-40s were not as resistant to colds as had at first been feared. They were paid three shillings a day (this was increased to seven shillings or 35 pence in 1973). They received free board and lodging (and hankies) and the return cost of transport to and from the unit.

Curiously, the majority of volunteers never caught a cold. Some were used as controls and given only a placebo inoculation of harmless saline solution. Others were simply resistant to infection by the virus then being tested.

'Many volunteers enjoyed their stay so much that they came regularly,' Andrewes reports. They were not allowed to return, however, for at least six months. By 1960 the unit had been visited by 6,399 volunteers, 2,896 men and 3,503 women – 742 of these married couples who shared one of the flats. One volunteer, told on reaching 50 that she would no longer be needed, gave a false name, dyed her hair and reduced her age to get back in. Unfortunately, she was recognised and sent home in disgrace. Some of the regulars claimed to be, 'hooked on the virus habit'.

Volunteers remained isolated with their room mates for 10 days and saw the research staff or other inmates at a distance of 10 metres, so conversation on a windy day had to be loud. The first four days was a quarantine period to make sure they were not incubating a cold on arrival, then they were put to work and only allowed home when all symptoms had abated – if they were among the cold catching unfortunates. They were allowed to go for walks in the country or play outside games like tennis or golf, but fraternisation with anyone other than the room mate was impossible.

Inevitably, sex raised its head from time to time and the cross-infecting offenders were expelled abruptly without pocket money or their fare home. They were also black listed!

Volunteers received two hot meals daily, delivered without contact with the staff, and cooked their own breakfasts from food kept in a small room refrigerator. Each volunteer received a free bottle of beer, cider or stout daily but had to make do without television. Deck chairs were provided for them to enjoy the sun (when there was any sun to be enjoyed) because most volunteers came in the summer. This could have presented something of a problem because most colds occur naturally in winter.

People from all walks of life volunteered. There was even a burglar who, on the last night when the farewell party was in progress, toured the flats and collected a good haul. One woman who didn't go to the party was able to identify him and he was soon apprehended in the nearby town of Salisbury. Anyone who had a history of TB, sinusitis, hay fever or asthma was excluded. On arrival, the volunteers were X-rayed to check for TB and other conditions and some undiagnosed cases of TB were found. Despite all the precautions, about three per cent of 'controls' who received only a placebo also developed colds.

'The doctor and matron wear sterile masks and gowns which are renewed daily,' Andrewes writes. 'When the unit first started we had separate masks and gowns for each flat but much time was wasted in changing and we soon concluded that this was unnecessary.' It was the doctor's duty to count the number of 20 centimetre square hankies used by the volunteer the previous day.

After the quarantine period was over, the subject was taken to the lab to receive either a cold virus or a placebo, flat sharers, of course, receiving the same inoculate. The resulting colds were graded into four types: **Abortive**, all clear within 24 hours. **Mild**, using more than four paper hankies a day for two to four days. **Moderate**, symptoms of headache, malaise, fever perhaps with shivering and sweating and a duration of up to seven days. **Severe**, upper respiratory symptoms, fever, loss of appetite, prostration, headache, cough and nasal symptoms throughout.

For those who succumbed, symptoms started within 48 hours, though this varied according to the virus used. The researchers soon noted that many colds were initiated but they quickly aborted.

Sometimes, only one of the flat sharers got the cold and the other remained well. What is more interesting is that they didn't seem to cross-infect each other even though they were living in such close proximity.

There was another problem – 'spontaneous' or 'wild' as distinct from cultivated colds which were much more frequent in winter. Where did these come from? It was also observed that the cultivated colds were harder to induce in winter, though no one had the faintest idea why. In the October to March period, around a third of any intake got colds. In the warmer period from April to September, almost half the intake succumbed.

After 1956, it became possible to separate different cold-producing viruses so the work was making progress, helped in part by research in the US and elsewhere. At first, the newly identified viruses could not be cultivated easily or even used to infect any convenient animal.

Most of the agents found so far by electron microscopy had proved to be tiny rhinoviruses. Now most viruses are inactivated by heating to 56 degrees centigrade for 30 minutes but they can survive at temperatures as low as -76 degrees for years. They can live for three days at 4 degrees but up to 27 days at -10 degrees.

The research was now proceeding all over the world and more and more viruses causing upper respiratory infection were being identified. In 1955 a new 'family' of viruses were discovered in the adenoids and tonsils, adenoviruses. These produced symptoms quite distinct from the common cold – fever and sore throat – and had a longer incubation period. It was soon discovered that adenoviruses could cause cancer in hamsters so human trials were quickly stopped even though there was no evidence that the virus caused cancer in human populations.

We now know, of course, that cancers can be transmitted by viruses though these almost certainly require an additional 'trigger' in the host to make them actively malignant.

Then the four parainfluenza viruses were found and it was discovered that these did not lead to long term immunity after infection, so reinfections were possible. In this case, after four days' incubation, symptoms similar to, but not as debilitating as, flu occurred.

During World War II in Britain, there was some interest in the concept of air hygiene, ironical but perhaps rational given the air pollution that was the inevitable product of total war. Disinfectant sprays and ultraviolet lamps were tested in schools as air purifiers in an attempt to limit the spread of upper respiratory infections as it was widely believed colds were transmitted by coughs and sneezes. Advertisements in London Underground trains constantly warned people to avoid spreading germs. The school tests proved fruitless, of course, but research continued at Salisbury into limiting the spread of dust that was found to carry bacteria, mainly streptococci rather than viruses.

Spreading infection from, for example, paper hankies was found to be no real problem. Transmission of colds by contaminated hands and other objects that were handled was 'unlikely to be very important'. Mixing infected people with the uninfected produced very few cases of cross-infection – in one test, of the 20 healthy volunteers, only one developed a cold and even that was suspected to be a 'wild' version.

To test the transmission of particles in the air, the researchers had their charges breathe, cough, sneeze and even recite Shakespeare with their heads in big polythene bags. The organisms recovered were then counted. At best 0.1 per cent remained suspended in air for any length of time and the rest fell to the ground. They could have saved a lot of taxpayers' money on those Underground ads.

Experiments with what was termed Coe virus (Coxsackie A21) produced 100 per cent colds in the inoculates but antibodies in the population generally were not developed. The virus was present in the nose of those infected but not evident in saliva to any extent. The researchers could induce infection by placing the virus in the nose or eyes but not so readily in the throat. It was rarely harmful if placed in the mouth. On drying, the virus quickly lost infectivity. And even with this virus, cross-infection was rare even when two people, one infected, shared a flat for a week or more.

So much for the ingrained idea of cross-infection which, as we will see in the next chapter, is still commonplace.

All this suggested to Andrewes and his crew that their volunteers were too resistant. What they needed – especially in the light of the Spitzbergen findings referred to earlier – was a nicely isolated community that had no immunity to cold viruses. Their eyes turned to the West Highlands of Scotland which was relatively warm but of low light intensity and where there were many isolated islands. The common cold there was regarded as a relatively serious illness and everyone was scared of encountering anyone with a cold.

Some years earlier, a small group of people had been isolated on Priest Island off the Scottish coast. After seven weeks without contact with anyone, these people were joined by the son of one of them who had a 'sniffle'. Within 48 hours, three of the party had succumbed to 'the most tremendous colds', far worse than those that occurred in normal life. In the light of this, Andrewes planned to isolate 12 people on Eilean nan Roan, the Isle of Seals, one and half miles off the coast of Sutherlandshire.

To cut a colourful story short, six infected volunteers failed to pass on a single cold to the 12 isolates either by cross-handling, droplet infection or sharing food preparation and meals. In desperation, a crofter who lived nearby and conveniently had a heavy cold was invited to spend 24 hours with the party because it was theorised that the laboratory induced colds of the six infectees had somehow lost transmissibility.

The isolates were divided into three groups exposed to different potential forms of cross-infection and 75 per cent of one group developed colds immediately. Obviously, a different virus for which they had no immunity was the cause but the researchers didn't at that time know that immunity to one cold virus did not give immunity to all sources of infection.

This led the team to ask: 'Is the transfer of an infective agent the whole story? Or is something more necessary to produce a cold?'

Next, a study of a small community, Bowerchalke, was implemented to learn more about the incidence and behaviour of colds in reality. The researchers found women have more colds than men, 'possibly because they are more exposed to infected children'. Colds were twice as prevalent where there were school age children, but not where there were pre-school infants only. Schoolgoers had more colds then adults but infants escaped unless the home also had schoolgoers.

Even then, the risk of cross-infection in the household was only one in five (20 per cent). Was this chance or good immunity?

Andrewes now tried to test the belief that chilling could induce a cold and he devised some rather harsh and uncomfortable ways of chilling his volunteers, including walking in the rain, getting soaked, then being placed in an unheated room to shiver for a while. The brave volunteers were all given a small dose of virus to make them susceptible but the shiverers failed to produce any colds between them. Andrewes was uneasy about this afterwards and wondered whether the failure to succumb was because they were 'not really stressed'.

Today, we would probably argue than a person who was totally convinced that a chill would precipitate a cold may well react accordingly because mental states can, we now realise, precipitate physical responses.

Other researchers, meanwhile, proposed that cold onset could not be explained by cross-infection because outbreaks seemed to occur in waves under certain climatic conditions and over a wide area simultaneously. Hence there developed a theory of latent viruses in all populations which were activated by environmental factors and, perhaps, inversely related to outside temperatures.

Andrewes concluded that bacteria and viruses are ever-present and constantly exchanged all year round. In this process, some could find an 'ecological niche' in a human host without inducing immunity, like *herpes simplex* which causes cold sores. The latest virus is then triggered into effect by some other factor. The problem with this was that successive colds in one sufferer were always produced by different viruses.

The research focus was now on the rhinovirus. In lab tests there were problems until it was discovered that cultivated viruses would grow well if three conditions were present: Low temperature, an acid medium, and rotation or movement of the cultures. The rhinovirus was also more difficult to handle because it was one of the smallest of all viruses.

So what of immunity? The team looked for antibodies in human blood serum. They found most volunteers who had no antibodies for a particular virus quickly developed them after infection with that agent provided a cold was induced. This proved that the viruses were of distinct 'races' or serotypes and that immunity had to be developed against each one.

This work continued at Salisbury until 1970. The idea of finding a simple cure for the common cold was long gone now that the family of viruses had been identified. A marked similarity between the rhinovirus and the virus known to cause foot and mouth disease in cattle was also noted. They learned that swallowed rhinoviruses could not produce immunity without cold symptoms. And now there was a long list of 89 serotypes to work with! All hopes of a single vaccine were abandoned.

This was not the case, however, with flu. It was learned than only one variant of influenza A was in circulation at any one time throughout the world, eventually to be replaced by a new form. So here it was possible, as we now know, to develop a vaccine though the work was long and slow. Rhinoviruses, unlike influenza A, co-exist at all times.

In 1960 a new virus was obtained from a schoolboy with a cold which proved readily transmissible but unidentifiable. In 1965, this virus – which was clearly different from the rhinovirus and produced different symptoms with a longer incubation and shorter duration – was also found in a student in the United States. It was larger than a rhinovirus and inactivated by ether. The electron microscope showed the schoolboy's variant and that of the American student were almost identical and more like a flu virus. They had a head or crown so were named coronaviruses. Little of this was known to Andrewes, however.

Research switched to the production of a live vaccine to combat flu and everyone, even the Russians, got into the act for here at last was something that could be patented and used commercially.

The files of the Common Cold Research Unit contain hundreds of letters from people who recommended all sorts of infallible ways of preventing or curing colds. None were backed by any worthwhile scientific evidence though there was some professional interest in two ideas: that antihistamines or vitamin C may be helpful.

The antihistamine idea led to wide commercial interest and huge pharmacy sales, especially in the United States but a review of the scientific literature by the Salisbury team made them very sceptical. There was no real evidence of any efficacy for either strategy. A Nobel prizewinner, Professor Linus Pauling, however, rekindled the vitamin C controversy when, in 1970, his book *Vitamin C and the Common Cold* was published. He recommended what came to be termed 'megadoses' of vitamin C in tablet form to head off or mitigate a cold – up to seven grams a day.

Still sceptical, the Salisbury team set out to test this proposition and gave some of their volunteers up to three grams daily by mouth for three days before inducing a cold by inoculation with a rhinovirus. Controls were given a similar looking placebo – so 24 subjects got vitamin C and 26 the placebo but all were given the virus. Nine colds developed in each of the two groups, which was a nice tidy research outcome. No correlation with any protective effect for vitamin C was found (for reasons that will become obvious later in this book).

Pauling, unfazed by this finding, blamed it on the use of cultivated rhinoviruses at Salisbury which were different from 'wild' viruses but Andrewes denied there was any evidence to support this. Pauling also said the dose was too low.

The possibility of developing a general antiviral agent that functioned in a similar way to antibodies was frustrated because a virus only exerts its effect when growing within a living cell. Any antiviral agent would have to be able to halt viral multiplication without disturbing the normal cellular processes. Another problem was the very short incubation period of rhinoviruses, unlike, say, measles or smallpox where development occurred much more slowly. So it was decided that prophylaxis was the only way to go, not cure.

At the end of the book, Andrewes finally poses some – but not all – of the questions that really concern us now:

- Some people never get colds. Why?
- Colds are very rarely troublesome in summer. Why?
- Is it a fact that some kinds of stress turn a harmless association with a virus into active disease?
- If so, just what are those stresses, how do they act, and can we counteract them?

For all that he was immersed in cold research for so many years, Andrewes never really got to grips with the concept of immunity. One could today shoot some big holes in the methods of the Salisbury research team but they were probably par for the course in their time. Scientists do science rather more precisely today.

What they did achieve was a solid base of hard information on which we are now able to build much more creatively to come up with the answer.

CHAPTER 3

TABLETS AND OTHER TREATMENTS

A popular family magazine recently published an article offering some 'hard facts' about colds, observing that, while we can send a man to the moon, there's still no cure for the common cold. Setting aside the economic idiocy of sending a man to the moon when half the world was impoverished or starving, the article was notable for the way it which it marshalled the myths and misstatements that invariably saddle the cold with a lot of unnecessary baggage.

After observing, correctly, that you can't catch cold by getting your feet wet or going to bed with wet hair, the author asserts the source of the cold is physical contact with a germ. If he is naive enough to think that all of us are not constantly assailed by, and exposed to, a vast array of exotic bugs in everyday life, the author is surely missing the point. He is persuading his readers that colds come from someone and somewhere else. By doing this he is wrongly focusing on the bug rather than the failure of the immune system.

His view of the cold is one in which you pick up a telephone used by an infected workmate and, bingo, you're going to get that cold whether you like it or not. But this is not true – and the reasons for rejecting such a simplistic and ill-conceived view will be set out in detail later in this book.

So what can the reader of this article do to protect him or herself from infection? Hygiene. Wash your hands, especially if you've touched anything that might harbour a germ. Having spent most of the day in the bathroom, carefully turning off the taps afterwards which your germ laden hands had previously turned on, and using once more the door handle, still infested with your bugs, you head off back to the wide world of rampant infection. That computer keyboard? The telephone? Oh, my god, quick, back to the bathroom...

There's no reason for not washing your hands or refusing to shake hands with someone, if that is your preference, but the farce of imagining you can reduce the incidence of colds by ardent hand washing leaves something to be desired in terms of health theory.

The author points out that it may be rude to rush off and wash your hands after some personal contact so the advice is to avoid touching your face for an hour or so until the viruses dry up and drop off your skin. No comment.

Finally, we get down to the immune system, which is to be kept tuned up with regular moderate exercise – okay, there's not much wrong with that in principle though some of the healthiest people I've known who lived to a great age never took a day's exercise in their lazy lives. A diet rich in fruit and vegetables, lots of sleep and stress beating relaxation therapy, the plan continues.

But what if this health promoting strategy fails and you *do* succumb?

The proposed remedy is to visit the local pharmacy and head for the aspirin or Panadol if you're aching and sore. Symptom relief is the object here. Cold suppressants and decongestants to relieve the dripping or congestion. The author advises against finding a physician to prescribe antibiotics because they don't work against viruses. Fair enough, but streptococci produce cold symptoms, too, and this could put certain people with specific risk profiles at even greater risk unless one knows for sure what agent is responsible for the symptoms.

Then megadoses of vitamin C are considered. 'But', says the author, 'while it has plenty of supporters, its efficacy is yet to be proven to most scientists.' Especially those sufficiently educated to know already that this doesn't work and can be dangerous for anyone with a predisposition to gastric problems and excess acidity. You could try garlic. If nothing else, that should keep personal contact down to a minimum.

The concluding paragraph says it all: 'Prevention is the best medicine. If you aspire to perfect hygiene and live the nutritionally sound, fit lifestyle we all dream of, you might avoid a visit from the rhino virus (sic) family this year.'

Sounds more like a nightmare.

As a contrast to this superficiality and the obvious inconsistencies, consider a report from the *Journal of International Medical Research* (March/April 1995). Italian researchers followed the ups and downs of 60 athletes for a three month period of intensive physical activity. Now these athletes, you may say to yourself, must be really fit. No common colds for them. Well, you'd be wrong. As a consequence of their efforts, they all managed to deplete their immune systems.

'There was also a significant decrease in natural killer cells (the good guys of the immune system)', the article states. The scientists were convinced that larger studies should be undertaken to examine the clinical significance of these findings.

There is a growing interest in the effects of exercise on the immune system. This seems to indicate that moderate exercise may activate the immune system, up to a point. But high intensity training is, 'currently considered able to induce an immune derangement making it easier to contract an infectious disease'. The athletes' problems could be a combination of performance stress and physiological demand, at least for some of the 'elite'. The simple fact is that after a single exhausting exercise session there is temporary depression of the immune response.

For the athletes, particularly those with demanding travel schedules as they compete in different countries with little chance of rest and relaxation in between contests, those responsible for their wellbeing are now evaluating the possibility of drug intervention to sustain immune function.

When grandmother told her charges to 'go to bed with a hot lemon and honey', she was probably a lot nearer the mark than the next generation of parents who headed for the medicine cupboard. The lemon, of course, is a potent source of vitamin C (provided it is freshly picked). Honey, as any committed herbalist will insist, contains all sorts of nutritional goodies like vitamin E. These vitamins may do you no good but they are unlikely to do you any harm, either. As a source of natural sugar, and an energy resource, it's a quick way to get a nutritional shot in the arm. More to the point, the honey offsets the acidity of the lemon and reduces some of the uncomfortable consequences for the digestive system. Above all, a hot sweet drink is relaxing and consoling, especially if you *believe* it's going to do you good.

The third strand of Grandma's advice was rest. In theory, rest allows the immune system to go to work unchallenged by other physical demands. Besides, you feel lousy so why not just sleep it off? Nothing wrong with that in principle. However, I knew an old man years ago who insisted that if ever he felt he was 'coming down with something' he would head for the garden shed, grab a spade and start digging frantically to work up a 'really good sweat'.

Now this wasn't as stupid as it sounds.

First, he was elevating body temperature and enhancing the physical conditions under which the immune system functions best. Second, he was increasing his metabolic rate, the rate at which body processes were functioning, and this may well have had the effect of getting his immune system onto the job faster and more efficiently. Anyway, whatever the scientific view, it seemed to work for this old bloke and he was never to my knowledge laid low and forced to his bed by any wayward bug. He had a positive and practical attitude to life and lived his natural term in full, popping off neatly enough with a fatal stroke when he was done.

The aspirin/paracetamol response of later generations requires more detailed comment.

Aspirin in its many forms is a wonder drug. First, it is an antipyretic. That is, it has the capability of reducing an abnormal body temperature or curbing a fever. Perhaps its greatest attribute is in relieving pain and easing swelling in inflamed tissues, especially in conditions like rheumatoid arthritis. It is an effective analgesic, in other words. Low doses of aspirin taken after a heart attack or stroke can prevent another occurrence. It is a blood thinner, cheaper than warfarin by far, but in some uses just as effective. It may be effective for pre-eclampsia in late pregnancy. Aspirin is used in ointments to treat some skin conditions or relieve inflammation and it even works (as Whitfield's ointment) to control tinea, particularly what is commonly termed athlete's foot.

One condition aspirin doesn't help much is the common cold.

The sceptic here will assert that aspirin, used while in the worst throes of a cold or flu, relieves the symptoms dramatically. The temperature comes down, the headache is relieved and so on. The problem is that aspirin also prolongs the suffering – you exchange a short sharp hit while the immune system gets itself together for a longer slow struggle back to normality.

By reducing body temperature, aspirin is counteracting a necessary function of the immune system. High temperature and fever are part of the healing process, a condition in which the good guys of the immune system can attack and destroy the invading pathogens and deal with them quickly. We'll look at immunity in a more scientific way later.

Suffice here to point out that relieving the cold/flu symptoms comes at a price. Aspirin is believed to reduce the level of vitamin C in the body just at a time when optimum levels are most needed. By thinning the blood, and what is termed antiplatelet action, it may well act in ways we do not yet understand to inhibit other aspects of the healing process.

Derived originally from the bark of willow or poplar trees around 1829, aspirin was first synthesised as salicylic acid in Germany in 1860 and proved one of the winners of drug manufacturer Bayer. Wonder drug it may still be (its healing properties have been known for centuries), but there are potential problems with use, especially for children under 12 years of age. The drug is also problematic for anyone with kidney or liver disease, a stomach condition, haemophilia, or about to undergo surgery. Sufferers from hay fever or asthma should not use it. Anyone taking medications for high blood pressure or being treated for congestive heart failure must avoid it. And it should not be used by anyone taking one of the other NSAID group of drugs because they, too, are blood thinners.

The tablets range in dose from 100 milligrams up to 650 though most seem to come in 325 milligram tablets today. When I was young, two 100 milligram tablets were the dose for cold sufferers. Today, people still opt for two (325 milligram) tablets but they're getting more than three times the dosage (650 milligrams). For young children with fever, there is a small risk, but a risk nevertheless, of liver failure.

To summarise: Aspirin has many important uses, especially as it is cheap and well tolerated by all but the very young and the elderly. But it does not have a part to play in treating the common cold, or the flu variants.

So what about paracetamol?

Paracetamol is an aspirin substitute that is less likely to have harmful side effects while lowering body temperature and relieving pain. Unlike aspirin, however, there is no anti-inflammatory action so it cannot control swelling or joint inflammation.

Paracetamol has been around in medicine's armoury since the last century but did not come into production for common use until after World War II. The prohibitions are broadly the same as those for aspirin though the dosage can be higher, 500 to 1000 milligrams every four to six hours. In all, a relatively harmless addition to the household medicine cupboard but of little use for treating the common cold unless, once more, you want to prolong the discomfort unnecessarily.

By now we have made it clear that any antibiotic drug has little part to play in a normal cold. There are some bacterial infections that may be threatening for young children or the elderly but use then is a matter for careful medical assessment.

The real goal is to develop the efficiency of the immune system. Unless the child's immune system is given an opportunity to identify and create antibodies for the many cold viruses, temporary or lifelong immunity cannot be conferred. Many pharmacologists, now worried by the rising resistance of the bad bugs to antibiotics, also fear that a child given an antibiotic for every wheeze or sniffle will not develop an effective immune system. So, unless there are indications of real threat and not vague considerations of indemnity, the sensible approach is to let nature take its course until something goes wrong.

Part of the problem is that anxious parents rush slightly sick children to the physician's surgery and expect treatment. Telling them to go home and give the victim hot lemon and honey and an early night tends to suggest nonchalance. The parent wants firm and decisive action to slaughter this bad bug and a prescription for an antibiotic has a nice aggressive ring to it.

Physicians could even prescribe a placebo (harmless non-drug tablets or medicines) when they know it is not in a child's interests to receive an antibiotic. But think of the outcry if a child given a placebo died from some undiagnosed condition. Anxious parents of sick children are not always rational about their fears.

According to the World Health Organisation's journal *Drug Information* (Volume 8, 1994), two thirds of all three year olds in the United States had received a dose of paracetamol or another proprietary medicine for a cold or a cough in the 309 days before a survey of 8,000 pre-schoolers was carried out.

Researchers concluded that proprietary cold medicines have no discernible beneficial effects. In fact, such medicines may be a home hazard causing poisoning and other accidents. They also pointed to a lack of information for parents on the proper use of home medicines. In the United States, more than $2 billion a year is spent on 800 or more products to ease cold symptoms. The WHO believes far more professional advice is required from pharmacists at the point of sale.

The whole picture is confused by rogue bacteria.

Many of the sore throats and other relatively minor but often uncomfortable inflammatory conditions can be caused, as we saw earlier, by streptococci or other bacterial agents. These are treatable with antibiotics, though that doesn't mean they should be so treated. The same principles of immunity, and the building of the body's defences, apply here though in a different form. Long term immunity is not created as antibodies are developed.

Rather, the level of resistance is raised to a point where the potential effects of the invading micro-organism are either negated altogether or minimised to the point where they give little discomfort. Each new encounter with that pathogen further strengthens the defensive response of the body.

If an antibiotic is prescribed, this resistance building is short-circuited and the prospect of future infection and troubling symptoms remains. Add to this the view of the World Health Organisation that the antibiotic era may already be in irreversible decline.

A lot of nonsense is talked about the 'sore throat'.

Any inflammation, as is true about a raised body temperature, indicates that the body is at war with an invader which it is seeking to deactivate. A sore throat, probably supported by swollen and tender glands in the neck, is an indication that the body is doing the job it was designed to do. It does not mean you are sick, just that you are avoiding sickness by putting up a fight.

If you start swallowing aspirin or paracetamol at this stage, all you will do is slow down the process and inhibit the function of the immune system. All too often this is done to prevent more serious infections or complications like pneumonia. However by prolonging the initial immune response, you are increasing the likelihood of wider infection.

This 'war' is fought at two levels, the physical and the psychological.

If, when the immune system properly reacts to an invading force, you fly into a panic. 'Oh my god, I'm getting a cold... But I can't, I'm getting married (competing in the final/going for that job interview/seducing my secretary) in a few day's time, I can't get a cold now...' Implicit in this response is a conviction that you're going to succumb, which probably ensures that you will because the mind, spurred by fear, has a powerful ability to determine physical outcomes.

If you took the other tack and said, when your throat feels sore and the glands swell: 'That's terrific. My immune system is on the job and because of that I know I'm not going to get that cold/flu/unidentified bug that's getting everyone else...', you'll have the very best chance of avoiding the outcome. Here the immune system is spurred by the expectation of a positive outcome.

So far we have been using broad generalisations to set the scene for some more detailed cold prevention strategies later. One other general point has to be made now. At the beginning and end of life, the levels of natural resistance, the ability of the immune system to identify, locate and terminate an invading pathogen, are less than in the period from, say, 12 years of age to, say, 65. At either end of the age spectrum, in other words, we are more vulnerable to attack – and because of this our medical care requires a more precise assessment of risk and treatment options.

There are other circumstances that can have a bearing on immunity – a lengthy stay in hospital, the aftermath of a serious disease, the use of some medications, particularly for inflammatory conditions, which undermine the function of the immune system, periods of sustained negative stress, death of a family member, and the like. There are times in anyone's life when they are more vulnerable to infection than usual. At these times, the conscious support of immune function is important once one realises that a point of vulnerability has been reached.

How this should be done will be detailed later.

Flu vaccinations are another sore point. Earlier we listed those people considered most at risk of flu who are generally regarded by the medical profession as first in line for the available vaccines. Two comments.

First, in an ordinary year when an epidemic is unlikely, there is little value in exposing elderly patients to the additional risk of vaccination. Only in circumstances where a powerful new strain is circulating is the need for vaccination clear and incontrovertible. Apart from that, it's a decision for the medical adviser who will be aware of the particular range of risk factors that affect the patient. To view a flu jab as similar to swallowing a vitamin tablet is probably unwise and a waste of valuable vaccine.

Second, flu jabs are not 100 per cent effective. Around 80 per cent of people receiving them will be protected wholly, or to the extent that any resulting infection by that particular form of the flu virus will be mild and enhance immunity for the future. If a virulent new strain appears suddenly, as it is more likely to do in these days of jet travel and mass tourism, the appropriate vaccine may not be available in sufficient quantities to meet demand. Too many people assume, because they have been inoculated against one form of flu, that this will somehow magically confer total immunity from all forms of flu. That is not so.

Conventional wisdom offers a mine of misinformation about the common cold, hence the purpose of this book. This is compounded by the general acceptance of redundant or misleading ideas about colds and how they are 'caught'. Until the emphasis turns from the threat of outside agents, the beguiling 'germ theory', to the idea that we live in a world crowded with competing organisms and micro-organisms all fighting for living space and sustenance, we will not have an adequate theory of cold prevention.

No matter how meticulous personal hygiene or even whether we lock ourselves in a sterile room for the rest of our lives, we will never escape the pathogens. What we must do is enable our defences to operate at full power and to develop that function in the frailer bodies of our children. The conceptual shift we have to make is to locate responsibility within the body, not without.

Unfortunately, medical opportunism, commercial vested interests and the fear mongering of some sections of the mass media, generate a false consciousness of many health related matters – drug use, cholesterol levels, nutrition, animal fats, alcohol, and many other aspects of everyday life.

The other day I watched an old man with osteoporosis walking with difficulty in front of my car. In one hand he held a carton of skimmed milk emblazoned with the symbolic image of a running athlete. In the other, he had a plastic pack of margarine. No doubt he doesn't eat eggs, either, for fear of elevating his 'cholesterol'.

Osteoporosis is a condition in which the bones thin and become brittle. A deficiency of calcium reaching the bones, perhaps because of poor nutrition or because of hormonal or deprivational factors like the female menopause or lack of sunlight lead to this condition. In children, the condition is known as rickets. It was relatively common in some British industrial cities, particularly in the north of the country, in the wake of the industrial revolution when rapid growth of urban factory employment combined with poor living conditions and diet. Not only was calcium implicated but an essential hormone, vitamin D – the sunshine vitamin – played a key role.

The British Government introduced a scheme after World War II whereby every school student was supplied free of charge with a small bottle of milk daily. A similar scheme was operated for a while in Australia. The idea was to feed children sufficient calcium (but in full cream milk that had not been leached of nutritional value so processors could make added value higher margin products from the butter fat). Alongside this, a regime of mid-morning exercise in fresh air outside was designed to get them in the sun, when there was some sun.

The result was a generally improving standard of community health, which was in part a response to this school policy and otherwise the consequence of improving living standards as disposable income and prosperity rose.

But the old man with his skimmed milk and polyunsaturated margarine was a sad victim of a false and crudely commercialised consciousness that impinges on the diet, health and lives of millions of people worldwide. The egg, that amazing food which can be produced without slaughter, is the cheapest form of high protein in any supermarket. To build the marketing fortunes of the meat producers and the canned or frozen variants, the egg – like vitamin rich butter, which offers outstanding nutritional value – had to be discredited as 'unsafe' or 'unhealthy'.

Contrary to popular belief, butter is a healthy food as many people are beginning to discover once more. The humble egg not only represents a much more efficient use of environmental resources but is an easily digestible whole food with some excellent nutritional properties. There is even a suspicion in some of the scientific literature that polyunsaturated fats may inhibit the functioning of the immune system.

Anyone who wants to manage their health competently needs to reassess some of the deceptions of our recent 'propagandist' past.

Current medical and nutritional research shows that full cream milk has only a low fat content, around 4 per cent. Animal fats appear to have no significant effect on serum cholesterol levels. Likewise the egg with its rich stores of vitamins D and E. White bread is no less nutritious than indigestible wholemeal. Red wine, in moderation – up to three to five glasses a day depending on sex, body weight and regular use, and preferably with food, is health giving, especially for anyone with a heart condition or high blood pressure. Red wine reduces oxidisability and LDL cholesterol whereas white wine has the opposite effect.

The only unimpeachable campaign of censure, that against the cigarette, is borne out by recent research and even then pipe and cigar smoking are not seen as harmful to the same extent, if at all in moderation. Cigarette smoking clearly is detrimental to health and the functioning of the immune system. It damages the upper respiratory system in particular, though the worst effects come from additives rather than the nicotine.

We're even discovering that the prohibitions on recreational drug use may have gone off the rails by banning the production of one of the earth's most useful fibres, hemp. Because of an irrational fear, based on misinformation, we are unable to prescribe two invaluable drugs for medical use – marijuana and heroin. The former is a relaxant with a variety of applications and the latter could greatly enhance pain-control options for the terminally ill. Instead, we have to use harsher opiates like morphine which, as any army medical orderly will tell you, is a rough old drug that just happens to be legal.

All this is not as far removed from the tribulations of the common cold as you may think.

In these days of political correctness, it is almost sacrilegious to criticise the conventional wisdom of health and nutrition. Yet, unless we sort out the truly healthy practices from the chaff of commercial or interest group motivated deceptions, we will not be able to put in place all the building blocks we need to end the scourge of the common cold.

CHAPTER 4

HOW THE IMMUNE SYSTEM WORKS

This will be a simplified account of the immune process, as far as is practicably possible. Anyone who wants to delve deeper should look at *Immunology* (1992) by Professor Janis Kirby, Professor of Biology at San Francisco State University, which should be available in any good library.

Kirby divides an immune reaction by the body into two interrelated functions – **recognition** and **response**. The immune system, she says, is able to discriminate between foreign molecules and the body's own cells and proteins. Once a foreign organism is recognised, the immune system enlists the participation of a variety of cells and molecules to mount an appropriate response and eliminate or neutralise the invader.

The invading organism has first to get through physical barriers like skin and mucous membrane. These provide an effective barrier to entry by most micro-organisms. Intact skin prevents the penetration of the majority of pathogens and also limits bacterial growth because of a low pH factor from the content of lactic and fatty acids. To gain entry, most pathogens need to colonise and penetrate the mucous membrane barrier, but this is inhibited by a number of defences. Special cells sweep attacking micro-organisms from the respiratory and gastrointestinal tracts.

All this is reassuring.

Saliva, tears, and mucous secretions 'wash away' invaders with antibacterial and antiviral proteins that destroy the pathogens. If the bad bug evades this first line of defence, there are other and bigger guns waiting.

The next line of physical barriers includes temperature and pH levels, and various soluble factors like naturally produced interferon. Chickens, for example, display an innate immunity to anthrax because of a high body temperature. Gastric acidity is a major barrier to infection. Few ingested micro-organisms can survive the low pH of the stomach. Interferon is derived from virus infected cells. Among its many functions is to bind nearby cells and induce a generalised antiviral state.

Immunity may be **innate** or **acquired and specific**, the latter reflecting the presence of a functional immune system which can recognise and selectively eliminate foreign micro-organisms and molecules. Unlike innate immunity, acquired immunity displays specificity, diversity, memory and the ability to recognise self or non-self, which is vital to prevent autoimmunity (when the system attacks itself). The immune system can recognise billions of uniquely different foreign antigens, it *remembers*. A second encounter produces a heightened state of immune reaction. Hence, lifelong immunity can be produced to counter many infections.

The innate and acquired immune system functions are orchestrated and mediate each other's response.

There are two major groups of cells in the immune system – antigen producing cells, B-lymphocytes, which mature within bone marrow, and T-cells produced by the thymus. These 'producers' are supported by the lymphoid organs – lymph nodes, the spleen, mucosal associated lymphoid tissue (MALT) or what we generally term 'the glands', and the tonsils, appendix and Peyer's patches.

Lymphocytes are extremely sensitive to X-rays. It may well be that with removal of the tonsils/adenoids, appendix and in some cases the spleen, even poorly shielded X-ray exposure, could have an effect on levels of immunity, especially in the context of damage arising from exposure to nuclear contamination. (US nuclear scientists believe that the early [1945-1970] X-ray equipment used on women in the US, Britain and Australia, for example, could account for three quarters of all breast cancers.)

If one 'producer' is immobilised, its products may be replicated and the role taken over by another organ.

When any form of inflammation occurs, there is increased blood flow and capillary permeability, and the phagocytes go to war. These are the pathogen 'eaters'. The affected tissue becomes inflamed and engorged and rises in temperature. The fluid that accumulates in the infected area has a much higher protein content than usual, while the swelling and permeability aid the flow of white blood cells (lymphocytes) from the capillaries into the threatened area. Four enzyme systems are now called into the battle to constrict blood vessels and support the destruction and removal of the pathogens (any disease producing agent).

Though the immune system can discriminate between specific antigens (any invading agent that stimulates the production of antibodies), as we saw above, a single genetic mutation is sufficient to enable the invader to escape detection, thereby avoiding an effective immune response.

Acquired and innate immunity do not occur independently.

Cells of the phagocyte system, mainly macrophages, are closely involved in activating a specific immune response. At the same time, various soluble agents produced during the initial response augment the work of the phagocytes. For example, when an inflammatory response develops, the soluble mediators produced attract cells of the immune system. The immune response in turn regulates the degree of inflammation. Through the carefully regulated interplay of these two forms of immunity, the systems co-operate to eliminate the invader.

From this, you can see that inflammation, and likewise a high body temperature, *are not negative symptoms that must be treated and ameliorated*, but positive immune responses working to protect your body from debilitating attack. As such, they need *augmentation,* not inhibition.

There are five classes of antigen – **foreign proteins** (that produce allergic responses), **viruses**, **bacteria**, **parasites** like the one that causes malaria, and **funguses** (that can cause tinea or mouth ulcers, for example).

In *Virus Hunting* (1991) by Dr Robert Gallo, there is an account of the discovery of this extended family of pathogens. Last century, Augustino Bassi, regarded as the father of medical microbiology, first identified a microbe (a fungus). By 1839 Johann Schonlein had linked a disease to a microbe, another fungus. Then Robert Koch, Louis Pasteur and others identified the microbial causes of most of the major diseases of the period.

In 1865 Pasteur pinpointed the first disease caused by a protozoan. By 1876 Koch had found the bacterium responsible for anthrax in sheep and, by 1882, had isolated the bacterium that caused tuberculosis. Pasteur went on to demonstrate that protection could be provided against some diseases by vaccination. The first virus, the tobacco mosaic virus, was found by Ivanovsky in 1892. Friedrich Loffler identified the virus that causes foot and mouth disease in cattle and the US army surgeon, Walter Reed, tracked down the virus that causes yellow fever.

While it was known by now that a virus could cause serious disease, it was not until the 1950s that scientists learnt to distinguish between RNA and DNA viruses. The RNA viruses were renamed *retroviruses* and we soon learned that they could cause some cancers as well as other diseases, though they were slow acting. By 1980, Gallo and his team had discovered the first cancer-causing retrovirus in humans. They went on to locate the human immunodeficiency virus, the forerunner to AIDS, which is also a retrovirus but in a new form.

In an updated edition of *The Body at War* (1993), Professor John Dwyer, an immunologist from the University of New South Wales in Australia, says viruses have developed far more sophisticated techniques for survival in the human body than have bacteria.

For a virus to grow and multiply, he says, it must enter into the sacrosanct environment of specific cells that will become unwilling hosts. Viruses are therefore parasites, living off other organisms. Viruses carry five to 200 genetic messages and a number of these are instructions for reproducing. In this way, a simple life form is capable of reproducing repeatedly, often damaging the host cell in so doing. Dwyer stresses that the infected cells have no escape from this role despite their defence mechanisms.

'The infected cell may die as it fills up with new viral particles and its membranes burst asunder as the virus explodes through the cell. So released, the virus simply moves into a nearby uninfected cell and another cycle is repeated. Even if a cell infected with a virus does not die, such damage can be done to the sophisticated control mechanisms which regulate cellular life that abnormal function and even a malignancy may develop – that is, a cancer cell may be born.

'In most cases, all that stands between us and domination by viruses is our immune system,' he says.

But Dwyer also points out that viruses are selective about host cells. The viruses that cause flu, for example, won't go near the kidneys and the herpes virus won't infect the liver. So viruses, too, are specialised and specific. Not only can viruses affect plants and animals, but they may also infect bacteria and this means a human bacterial infection could give a virus a piggy back ride into a host cell.

'Viruses are so specifically designed to invade one cell type that those causing animal diseases rarely infect humans, and vice versa,' Dwyer says. The influenza virus, for example, has a predilection for cells lining the human throat.

Bacteria, on the other hand, are complete life forms and not parasites, so they don't need an unwilling host to reproduce. But they are still very threatening to a human body even though they can live happily outside a host. Dwyer shows how bacteria, as they multiply in the body, may secrete toxins that disturb one or more body functions. They can invade tissue and multiply rapidly causing conditions like pneumonia. Surrounding tissue may get hurt in the counter attack launched by the immune system.

There are thousands of bacteria types, each with about 1000 genes which they can exchange with nearby organisms. When they encounter an antibiotic, for example, they mutate into new forms that resist the antibiotic. Most of the bacteria, Dwyer adds, that were killed by penicillin 50 years ago are now resistant because they have genes that produce an antidote. Because they reproduce so rapidly, bacteria can evolve significantly within a short time.

'It is very common', Dwyer explains, 'especially with babies who have antibiotic treatment for, say, a chest or ear infection, to solve one problem while creating another. While clearing up the ear infection, the antibiotics may also kill off the bacteria in the gastrointestinal tract. The result is that fungus (candida, more commonly called thrush) can spread up and down the intestinal tract.' Dwyer speculates that the immune system evolved among developing species over hundreds of millions of years and adapted many times to counter new survival modes adopted by microbes. Before birth, the growing foetus retraces these evolutionary steps. The developing thymus gland becomes the control centre of the immune process and begins to produce vital T-cells. But, because the human body, like all species, is designed to self-destruct, the thymus gland works hard only for the first few years of life until there are sufficient T-cells to meet the needs of a normal life span. *Then it shuts down.*

Once all our T-cells have been used up, we have reached our use-by date.

T-cells, however, are a primitive form at an early stage of evolution. Antibodies later evolved to increase the complexity and effectiveness of the immune response. This is where the B-lymphocytes come into the picture. These give us the capacity to produce antibodies to counter a vast range of antigens. They take up residence in the lymph nodes, the sites of most of the major immunological battles, and wait there until an enemy tries to pass. Their lifecycle is relatively short compared with the T-cells so they are constantly replenished by bone marrow output.

During pregnancy, a mother's immune system works diligently to top up antibodies against potential antigens likely to be encountered by the baby after birth. These last for about three months by which time the growing child has the ability to produce its own antibodies and, provided unnatural processes do not interfere (like bottle feeding), everything should flow smoothly to provide the baby with an effective immune system. Unfortunately, hospital care in the first few days may expose the baby to antigens that have found a niche in that environment but have not been encountered by the mother's immune system before or during pregnancy. So, for the child, there may be no immunity to attack by these organisms (termed nosocomial infections).

Breast milk provided in the first few days of the baby's life, colostrum, contains high levels of antibodies to top up the child's immunity and, even after the milk flow is fully established, antibodies are passed to the suckling child. After six months, these levels fall significantly. So enhanced are the immunological properties of breast milk that it can even be used as eye, ear or nose drops for minor infections, Dwyer says.

There's a lot more to the process of developing immunity than that.

We haven't for example, even touched on the role of the NK cells, probably the ancestors of the T-cells and also resident in the lymph nodes. These, it seems, may be particularly important in preventing cancers because cancerous cells cannot be removed by antibodies. Dwyer also notes a connection between NK cells and various psychological factors related to stress.

Dwyer, incidentally, asserts that most cancers cannot be put down to viral infection. 'This puzzle', he says, 'only started to take better shape with the recent and most puzzling discovery that oncogenes can be found in normal human cells not infected with viruses.' This suggests that this may be an essential part of the 'programming' of cells to self-destruct when our time is up.

'Cancer could be seen as nature's final solution to the hazard that is longevity', he adds. The work is developmental and there are many uncertainties and inconsistencies.

Where the virus seems to play a role is in carrying a cancer activating signal, thereby inducing cancer following the invasion of a cell by that virus which either has its own oncogene or one received from a previously infected cell. Another trigger mechanism is where the control mechanism of an oncogene is disrupted by external environment factors, like the X-ray, contamination with asbestos or any chemical that can interfere with DNA structure.

This gives some idea of the complexity of the bodily responses underlying the common cold and the requirements of any strategy to prevent infection.

Though the immune system has clearly evolved to carry out an amazing task, total defence, the hostile organisms, too, are evolving and constantly searching for a chink in the immunological armour. For that reason, preventing infection means one must create the most favourable conditions possible for the system to work well. This is where many people start to get bogged down in 'false consciousness'.

We have already seen that the vitamin enthusiasts are getting it wrong by focusing on parts rather than the whole.

The nutritional requirements of a healthy body, one that adequately supports a well tuned immune system, are both simple in chemical content and complex in interaction and interdependence. We talk of swallowing vitamin C tablets, iron supplements or even vitamin D pills with little idea of how these chemicals interact with everything else that involves the body, internally and externally. Instead of resorting to a nutritious fruit like an orange, which offers a complex range of vitamins and fibres, even minerals, which are 'orchestrated' within the fruit itself and supported by fructose, a readily usable sugar, we talk of the orange purely as a source of vitamin C.

Pregnant women, or those who are iron deficient, for example, are advised to take slow release iron supplements. They may be given no information about the supporting need for vitamin B12 or vitamin C, and how these chemicals may be affected by exposure to sunlight as part of the necessary process of ingestion, synthesis and metabolism.

Coal miners, or people required to work for long periods without exposure to sunlight, soon become 'run down' and eventually sick. Yet, seduced by suspect propaganda, we are now denying many children adequate access to sunshine, let alone allowing the sun and light exposure to strengthen and harmonise, or co-ordinate, their growth and maturation.

Why, in this age of super science and space travel, are we so inept at preventing colds despite all the jogging and pseudo-healthy diets? We talk of being stressed and run down and see the need to 'recharge our batteries' by taking a holiday somewhere in the sun – but when we get there we don sunglasses, floppy hats with neck and ear flaps, sunblock lotions, long sleeves and baggy trousers and try to prevent as much light as possible from reaching our pale and deprived skins. And when next we succumb to a virus and get a cold or flu, or something worse, we wonder how it is that this can happen when we have such a healthy lifestyle.

The problem is, we don't have anything of the sort.

Viruses evolve and mutate, often quickly as we have seen, and the changing lifestyles of many people in the industrial or urban world can facilitate this process to our detriment. New pathogens slip past the highly sophisticated defence systems of the body, as they have done with several well publicised but contained epidemics in Africa in recent years. Poverty, malnutrition, overcrowding and misguided health care create the ideal breeding grounds for antigens that will not easily be recognised, even by the best functioning immune system.

Even in wealthy communities, a population that is deprived of the environmental necessities – light and sunshine, clean air, pure water, genuinely nutritious food – is threatened. We work for most of the daylight hours under restricted spectrum lighting (often in front of visual display units that produce poorly understood electromagnetic fields and questionable microwaves) and the combination cannot be termed 'healthy'.

Add to this the quirks, shortcomings and immune susceptibilities of individuals. Some may have had unusual childhood experiences or serious illnesses. Others were deprived of essential needs for a period. Some had parents with cranky ideas who inflicted all kinds of idiocies on them. Some, in the lottery of genetic patterning, fared badly and are destined to suffer serious illness. They just inherited the wrong traits. The foregoing demonstrates that the first task is to build, then maximise, immune potential.

Once that task is realised, the likelihood of succumbing to the common cold, or any antigen, is sharply reduced. Even then, that is only part of the story, the physical part. We have also to build into this protective strategy the function of the mind and see where psychology meets pathology. Without a healthy mind, a healthy body is hardly possible.

CHAPTER 5

MORE PIECES OF THE PUZZLE

No one factor, a quirk of fate, determines who gets sick. In the previous chapter we looked at the role of the immune system. It would be tempting, and too easy, to blame a failure of the immune system for whatever reason, or complex of reasons, for all illness.

Yet, in the basic way that some people approach health, there is a belief that by stuffing down a particular vitamin, or worse, a king hit of multivitamins, we will magically avoid viral and bacterial infection. The common cold, as we have seen already, cannot be warded off with megadoses of vitamin C in the way that vampires were once said to be diverted by garlic.

Let's move to a psychological view, especially as we have already linked immune failure with stress factors which are clearly mediated by the mind rather than the body. Blair Justice, in *Who Gets Sick* (1987), is convinced that our heads, or rather our minds, affect our health. For him, mind and body are parts of a functional whole regulated by the brain.

'Rather than losing brain cells as we grow older', Justice says, 'we can actually extend our neural connections – just as old rats become smarter and run mazes better. Both brain chemistry and structure are affected by the way we experience and perceive the environment.'

Mental processes, in this view, affect and moderate the physical – even at the most basic level. Something as simple as a sense of humour can play a role when the chain reaction of laughter stimulates the production of antibodies! (Just how one proves this is open to question.) Take a more concrete but controversial example. You experience the first symptoms of the onset of a cold and the resulting inflammation makes you feel uncomfortable. You think to yourself, 'I'm not going to get a cold at all, that is just my immune system doing the job. In a few hours, the battle will be won.'

Do you succumb to the virus?

Probably not, because your mental perception has reinforced the work of your immune system and you have not indulged in panic at what was happening. However, what would have happened had you reacted by saying to yourself, 'Oh my god, I'm coming down with a cold and I've got to do (such and such) tomorrow. This is an absolute disaster and I know I'm going to be out of action for a week now...' Chances are you're gone. You've convinced yourself, undermined the good work of your immune system and in effect lowered your guard or 'switched off' the battle that should have taken place. If you then rush into the kitchen and swallow three aspirin in a desperate attempt to snare the bug, you back up this negative mental reaction and the immune response by lowering your body temperature, reducing vitamin C levels, changing blood viscosity (thickness), etc.

So you go to bed with a beauty of a cold and all because you reacted badly.

A writer in the *New England Journal of Medicine* (Angel) observed back in 1985 that people who 'continue to believe simplistically in singular causes (viruses, genes etc) as sufficient to explain disease angrily charge that anyone who suggests that our attitude and moods contribute to whether we get sick is "blaming the victim" and implying the person "caused his own illness".'

How can the way we think affect our immune system?

It's like that 'gut feeling' some people are always talking about, Justice says. Body is a part, an inseparable part, of mind. His theory of illness is that the brain, the nervous and immune systems, and the endocrine functions are so closely linked that they form *a single regulatory network*. What happens in the mind, for example, may influence profoundly the process of DNA repair.

Justice is concerned that conventional medical practice remains wedded to a non-mind view of illness – he bluntly describes this as 'a mind-less concept of disease' – which is clearly limited and in many cases unhelpful. This is why, he believes, the outlay of twice as much on cancer research as on space research in the past 25 years has produced very little progress in preventing cancers.

Psycho-social factors can depress the function of the immune system. It's not the stresses or the bugs that kill us, Justice argues, but the way in which we respond to these assaults. This leads him to the view that 'positive attitudes and beliefs can protect and restore our health by turning on self healing systems'.

Now the last thing at this stage is for the reader to see a resemblance here with the 'positive thinking' of evangelist Norman Vincent Peale because the standpoint is very different. It is also much more partial because, as we see in later chapters, the strategy for ending the ravages of the common cold relies as much on the physical as on the state of mind, and the beneficial outcomes are dependent on a rational co-ordination of all these elements. So Justice is stating a valuable, but partial, case to counterbalance a major shortcoming in some current medical thinking and practice.

Charging into the pharmacy and rushing out with a bag full of antipyretics, pain killers, cold suppressants and vitamin tablets will do nothing to benefit a person's suffering other than *to relieve symptoms*. On the contrary, as we have seen already, some forms of treatment may even suppress or slow the functioning of the immune system and lengthen the time taken to get better.

Justice believes that our cognitions (thoughts, beliefs, attitudes) and the social support we perceive in our lives can alter the levels of our hormones and neurotransmitters, chemical messengers that carry on communication between our cells and largely govern the activity of many physical processes. His explanation of disease embraces mind, body and genetic predispositions, and environment.

'The more vulnerable we are, the more risk we run of getting sick', Justice says. 'The factors that place us at risk range from our attitudes and appraisals in coping with stress to the kind of food we eat and the genes we inherit.' This puts the balance between **risk factors** and **resistance resources** as the determinant of whether we stay healthy or fall sick.

There's a problem here, of course, because it falls short of an adequate explanation for the protection offered by vaccination where, clearly, the mind doesn't have much to do with the consequence. But it may go a way towards explaining why some people who are exposed to serious risk, high levels of nuclear radiation for example, seem to escape the likely consequences. A BBC television documentary dealing with the effects of nuclear radiation showed an interview with a Japanese resident of Hiroshima at the time of the explosion of the US atom bomb. While her two children died quickly of radiation sickness, and she suffered this herself, she survived and today appears, despite her age and emotional suffering, to be in good health.

Not only had she coped physically and philosophically with the physical injury she experienced and high levels of radioactivity, but she was also able to deal with the death of her children and the destruction of her environment. Few people are ever likely to suffer greater personal stress.

Stewart Wolf, a clinical researcher in medicine and physiology at Temple University, Philadelphia, sees disease as 'a way of life' – the end result of how people react to life's problems. In the case of the Japanese survivor of Hiroshima, he may have a telling point.

In *Sickness and Healing*, anthropologist Robert Hahn develops the concept of 'anthropological medicine' to take the place of what he calls the present bio-medicine because the causes of all sickness are both biological and cultural. All illness, in his view, is 'culture bound'. We'll return to this point later but suffice to say here that Hahn argues for the patient's subjective view of his or her illness to be incorporated in medical practice and theory. In other words, what one believes about illness has a profound effect on the nature of illness.

The mind/body hypothesis, however, concerns us here because most of the microbes that afflict us are already and always present in the body in one way or another. So other risk factors must have a role to play if we are to succumb and these probably include stress, or rather *negative* stress, and work or family conflict or dissatisfaction.

Robert Rose and his team at Boston University School of Medicine studied illness affecting 416 air traffic controllers for three years. About one fifth of the sample averaged more than five mild to moderate illnesses a year, mostly upper respiratory infections, asthma, viral diseases and gastrointestinal problems. Another 20 per cent had one episode or less a year. Those who were frequently sick had lower morale and expressed job dissatisfaction. They perceived more events in their lives outside work as 'stressful'. Given that the majority of all acute cases of illness are upper respiratory infections, mostly colds, *we don't have to catch a bug to get sick*. The pathogen is there waiting for the right time to strike when our immunity is in some way compromised. As Justice explains it, peaceful co-existence between micro-organisms – such as streptococci – and the human hosts is the rule while disease is the exception.

So what else can lower resistance, that is, impact on the functioning of the immune system?

Fatigue, poor nutrition, emotional distress, age, an inability to cope for psychological or health reasons, genetic traits – there are numerous possibilities which may act in concert with a specific viral assault to produce illness. Some physical stresses, for example, may be so overwhelming that mind, the psycho-social mediator, becomes irrelevant.

Justice argues, quoting from other scientific sources, that the brain uses neuroactive chemicals and their receptors, as well as electrical impulses, to establish a far reaching influence over a healthy body. This chemical 'behaviour' adjusts to changes we perceive in personal wellbeing as we deal with other people and situations. Every change we perceive gives rise to a host of questions:

- Can I handle this?
- What's going to happen if I can't?
- What response is possible?

Such thoughts produce, through the brain's neurotransmitters and neuroregulators, 'co-ordinated metabolic and cardiovascular alterations' that prepare us for action or retreat. Have you never experienced, for example, that chest tightening in the heart region when you are unexpectedly made aware of something that shocks you? For Justice, calling on the earlier work of Lionel Tiger in *Optimism: The Biology of Hope* (1979), this reduces to the idea that, if we see things as hopeless and decide to give up, that decision is dutifully conveyed by the brain to the body which proceeds to carry out the order.

Healthy people, he concludes, are distinguished by the way they look on their past and present difficulties and whether they view their lives as interesting, varied and relatively satisfying. By contrast, people who have frequent illnesses are likely to see life as threatening, demanding and frustrating.

Again, there are problems with this view.

Consider, for example, someone who has been treated repeatedly with an antibiotic, possibly the wrong one, for a run of ailments and as a consequence has failed to develop immunity by producing sufficient antibodies to the antigens. Without immune protection, this person is at much greater risk and, though this risk may be enhanced by their state of mind, the mental state may well have been affected or undermined by constant illness.

Drugs may also present a problem.

In *The Archives of Family Medicine* (April 1995) a case was reported of a patient on verapimil to control high blood pressure who had experienced repeated and prolonged viral infections. It was believed the drug had suppressed this patient's lymphocyte production and thus immune response. His body did not react normally to an influenza vaccine. In this case the verapimil dose was lowered and the patient's immunity appeared to return to normal. Malic and other researchers concluded that calcium channel blockers may 'transiently disturb immunoregulation'. Before you panic and flush your antihypertensive drugs down the toilet, this is only an opinion at this stage which requires much closer investigation.

However, the idea that attitudes, beliefs and moods affect the action of chemical messengers in the brain has greatly expanded our knowledge of how we can get sick or, more importantly, how we can stay well.

Justice argues: 'When we believe our problems are beyond control, another hormone – cortisol – increases and impairs our immune system, making us more vulnerable to infection and some cancers. When we think we cannot cope effectively, still another chemical messenger – dopamine, which is related to our sense of reward and pleasure – diminishes.'

He believes fast acting neural transmitters can excite or inhibit the receptors of the cells they contact. Hormonal 'messengers' in the blood stream are slower acting – they may take minutes or hours to speed up our natural cell metabolism and activity rate. A third group of messengers induce cells to grow in size and number and to differentiate. This activity is influenced by neurotransmitters and peptide 'messengers' like endorphins, which are able to enhance or diminish the actions of the messengers.

Suffice to establish here that there is another 'realm' of physiological and psychological action involved in all illness – that the body, the brain, the glands and the immune system connect and communicate by way of messenger molecules that are sensitive to thoughts and reactions.

So far, few of these chemical messengers have been identified – rather in the way that cold causing viruses had to be tracked down over many years – and even less is known of their orchestrating functions. They are certainly influenced by environment and genetics and their action and response can certainly be 'jammed', shut down, by drugs, viruses, bacteria, the wrong foods, defective genes, ageing or stressful situations and perceptions or beliefs.

Even the inherent 'natural drugs', the pleasure transmitters or pain killers, enkephalins and endorphins, were only discovered in 1975. We know little more than that they have a major role to play in sexual excitement and satisfaction, and must therefore play an important role in the whole reproductive process. The point at which this links with health, and psychological stability, opens up a Pandora's box of prejudice and culturally mediated beliefs.

Among these chemical messengers are the prostaglandins, the hormone like substances that play a part in the process of inflammation.

Producer cells rely on an enzyme, cyclo-oxygenase, to do their work and it is this that appears to be destroyed by the action of aspirin and the way in which it acts to inhibit inflammation. People who suffer from arthritis, for example, have high levels of prostaglandins. An excess can cause pain, inflammation and fever yet a certain level is needed for kidney function, digestion, reproduction and blood circulation. The prostaglandins are manufactured by almost every tissue in the body.

Here the plot thickens.

Certain foods may have a significant and rapid effect on mood, memory and attention span and can affect choice which feeds back into mood. Sweet foods, for example, may increase the output of serotonin in the brain and provide a calming effect. Too much sugar may release endorphins which, with serotonin, diminish sensitivity to pain – or even distress, which is emotional pain.

Justice reports that researchers were surprised to discover that the function of neurotransmitters in the brain could be enhanced by diet. High protein food increased alertness and concentration while carbohydrates promoted lethargy and relaxation. The response, of course, is mitigated by age and gender – so older people are more sensitive to these effects and women become calmer and more sleepy after eating carbohydrates than do men.

If you want to be calmer, try pasta which increases the tryptophan and serotonin in the brain. The tryptophan also makes one less sensitive to pain. Or, to produce the opposite effect, a meal of steak and eggs will increase tension levels and make you more alert. For some if not most people, a carbohydrate craving has more to do with the need for serotonin than with indulgence. Justice believes junk foods, high in fat as they are, can lead to impairment of the immune system, too.

Some foods may give pleasure by triggering the release of beta-endorphins, a form of peptide. They act on the brain in a manner similar to morphine and are the so-called natural opiates. These substances include the enkephalins (the least potent) and the dinorphins (the most potent) which were first identified only in 1975. Each has a different pathway in the brain and they are pharmacologically identical to narcotics. Morphine is addictive because it mimics the neural transmitters of the natural opiates.

There have been recent scientific attempts to trigger the flow of the natural opiates for procedures like dentistry. The use of transcutaneous electrical nerve stimulation or TENS instead of novocain to prevent pain is one possibility. A low voltage shock is administered and appears to offer anesthesia without side effects or needles.

There is some evidence that the key cells of the immune system have receptors for endorphins and enkephalins. Endorphins, as we have seen, are used by the body to relieve mental and physical pain. Good feelings, perhaps from a positive social encounter, may well depend on the natural opiates which are directly associated with 'happiness'. This reinforces the principle of a psycho-biological process involved in good health. The brain also produces valium like chemicals related to the endorphins – benzodiazepines – which quell anxiety, relax muscles and promote sleep.

Vitamins have long been implicated in the story of the common cold. When Linus Pauling dropped his bombshell on an already tired and suspect idea by claiming that megadoses of vitamin C could significantly influence susceptibility to and the severity of a cold, his reputation as a Nobel Prize winner for science caused people to think again. The manufacturers of the most popular 1 gram effervescent product claimed only that it would promote more rapid healing of injuries. There was a general belief that maintaining high blood serum levels of ascorbic acid would maximise immunity and compensate for the loss of natural vitamin C in food transportation and processing, and through cooking or other dietary factors. It was already widely known that heat destroyed this vitamin.

Thinking about vitamins, and their supplementation through

artificial means, was as primitive as many of the beliefs about the common cold. At least those people who opted for the much more expensive multivitamin and mineral supplements recognised the interdependence and interaction of these chemicals. What the users did not seem to appreciate was the extent to which vitamins in general, as one component of diet, constituted part of a much wider and more finely balanced system.

An analogy of a symphony orchestra has been used elsewhere but it is worth restating here.

The complex body processing of food, water, air and all the external sources of sustenance involving light, temperature, humidity and even social support requires the interdependence of these parts for the viable functioning of the whole organism. Simply pinpointing a small cog in this great wheel, vitamin C, or the vitamins A, D and E for that matter, is rather like building a working motor vehicle from three tyres and two seats. Without assembling all the necessary parts in a coherent and functional manner, the project is impossible.

To feel a sense of security as a consequence of taking a few vitamin C tablets is a red herring in the search for any lasting resistance to the common cold. A preferable strategy would be to take up the advice of that wise man who once asserted: 'You can buy more vitamins for a fraction of the cost in a fruit and vegetable store than you'll ever get from a bottle.' Or something like that.

Consider an observation.

An Australian family enjoys good health and no one ever gets a cold. This is attributed mainly to the fact that each member consumes before breakfast a tumbler full of fresh squeezed undiluted juice from local sun ripened oranges. Apart from this being a pleasant start to the day, it ensures the family members have their daily nutritional requirement, such as we understand it, of vitamin C. But this is ingested along with all the other constituents of the fresh orange – complementary vitamins, fructose which is preferable to sucrose (ordinary supermarket sugar), and the accompanying minerals and fibres dependent on local soil conditions.

It would be reasonable to argue that this breakfast routine is, indeed, beneficial to health but it would be drawing a very long bow to say that this is *the reason why* no family member ever develops (not catches) a cold. However, orange juice provides a few of the essential *resources* needed for sustaining good health.

In our strategy for ending susceptibility to colds, we are going to move well beyond such a simplistic view while maintaining the position that dietary factors, and the naturally created vitamins and minerals ingested from everyday foods, have a vital part to play.

An apple a day, or an orange for that matter, does not the doctor keep away. But it creates a frame of mind in which the eater recognises the relationship between fresh food and health, and between some conscious dietary decisions and wellbeing. Having said that, however, it must also be stressed that diet and nutrition is one of the most abused and deceptive areas of mass media speculation. Astute public relations firms achieve a great deal for wealthy clients by promoting the products that are profitable rather than the foods that are really beneficial.

We know that vitamin A also functions as a potent 'immune enhancer' but it is also believed that polyunsaturated fats inhibit the immune function.

Then there's garlic, much feared by English and other tourists on French trains. The Department of Pharmacology at Newcastle University is currently testing garlic to identify the beneficial effects when used in sufficient quantity. In an article in *The Australian Doctor* (14 April 1995) it was asserted that garlic is:

- Anticoagulant in effect four to six hours after use.
- Antihypertensive – diastolic blood pressure on one trial was shown to have been reduced by an average 10 per cent.
- Antimicrobial against E-coli and salmonella and other pathogens.
- Antibacterial, in some cases it could be as effective as an antibiotic.
- Antifungal, especially against Candida albicans.

This panacea, when added to tasty food and washed down with good red wine (in moderation) and followed by some fresh fruit and blue cheese made in the locality appears to give some French people an extraordinary level of freedom from heart disease. *C'est la bonne vie!* Perhaps the worthy researchers of Newcastle University should extend their terms of reference.

Having provided the body with the raw materials it needs to fashion rude health, we have to establish the other keys to immunity. And, even then, we have only tuned up one section of the orchestra, the strings.

The important point to grasp here is that any one deficiency, a failure to maintain appropriate levels of vitamins, minerals or other trace elements essential to a balanced system – within the quite wide parameters the body can tolerate – has to be corrected to get the orchestra playing in tune again.

Two other key sections of the orchestra are the circulatory and the hormonal systems. Consider two simplistic examples.

Many women, perhaps in early pregnancy or in some localities, are deficient in iron. This affects blood quality, the red cell content which, you may recall, is the other side of the coin to the white cell or lymphocyte content serving a functioning immune system. Men, too, may be iron deficient as are plants or other life forms under certain soil conditions. The simple but inadequate answer is to rush down to the pharmacy and buy a pack of iron tablets. There's a problem. Iron is not easily ingested and will simply be excreted if it is not taken with vitamin B12 and vitamin C to facilitate absorption in a user adequately exposed to daylight, or such as we know to date. There may be other more complex processes involved, too. Any attempt to deal with anaemia, iron deficiency, by simply swallowing an iron tablet is doomed to fail.

When people reach middle age, their hormonal balance changes.

Women, designed for reproduction, fare worst at this change of life because there may be a relatively sudden downturn in oestrogen output which brings about the symptoms we generally describe as the menopause. Accompanying this there are behavioural changes and, for some people, a profound change in feelings of wellbeing. By supplementing oestrogen, or counterbalancing oestrogen and progesterone, with tablets or slow release patches, most of these unwanted symptoms can be alleviated and the user 'let down slowly' into a more comfortable ageing process.

The human hormonal balance is acutely sensitive to any attempt at fine tuning yet some, usually male, medical advisers approach the subject wearing hobnail boots. Any attempt to interfere with such a delicately poised system requires a specific medical history of the patient, acquired from a careful interpretation of blood tests. That information must be related to every other health consideration that may interact with the readjustment of hormonal balance in what is, essentially, an unnatural process.

Any imbalance or disharmony of either of these systems may impact profoundly on health generally. Only one instrument, let alone a whole section, has to be out of tune for the orchestra to play badly.

Elsewhere we have considered, rather superficially, the misrepresentation of foods said to be 'healthy' for a variety of commercial or 'politically correct' reasons. Among some of the more colourful subjects of this propaganda are fish oil (just look what is does for the Japanese), wheat germ (why not eat the whole grain?), food fibre, and a range of herbal 'remedies' like evening primrose oil that may, or may not, offer any benefit to humanity. Such is public discontent with our present medical delivery system that people have turned in force to healers like naturopaths, chiropractors, and a whole host of (sometimes unqualified) alternative or complementary practitioners.

Depending on the state of mind or body of the patient, these service providers may offer solace or even a cure. But alongside this, many appear to offer some questionable propositions about health in general and diet in particular. Buyer beware, *caveat emptor*. A banal comment bears repetition here. Our medical system is illogical because we pay our practitioners to keep us sick, not make us well. Or put another way, if we only paid the practitioner when we were well, he or she would have a vested interest in keeping us that way. As things stand, the opposite applies. Anyone wishing to promote and maintain rude health would be well advised to by-pass food faddists, incoherent medical prophets and others who can be shown to gain from human misfortune rather than actively promote health.

As Dr Peter Baume observed in *The Australian Doctor* (12 May 1995), 'there are no good or bad foods, it's how we use them which is good or bad...' Or Dr A. R. P. Walker writing in the *Journal of the Royal Society of Medicine* (January 1995): 'Energy intake explains only a small proportion of cases of obesity, and sugar intake explains very little of the variance in dental caries, the same applies to salt intake and hypertension.'

One last aspect of the story so far needs to be revisited here: the genes we inherit from our parents. We are what the genes we inherit, or the viral mutations of damaged genes, determine. Following in the wake of the great gene study, an attempt to map the genetic structure of the whole human body and discover which gene does what and why and to whom, we have learned that many diseases, or susceptibility to infection or malfunction, is the consequence of a preprogrammed structure. Even body build, fatness or thinness, is ordained by inheritance.

In part, therefore, a functioning immune system is the inherited product of evolution and millions of years of human genetic refinement. Its effectiveness is directly affected by the lifestyle, environmental adaptations and even culture of our ancestors. This system, as we have seen, is all that stands between us and misery or death. For most people in urban industrial societies, it continues to function despite the burdens placed on it, no doubt adapting along the way.

Medicine in the future may well devise forms of genetic control, manipulation or correction that will remove the threat of certain diseases in a way parallel to the mastery of TB, smallpox or polio by vaccination.

Because of scientific medical discoveries like the antibiotic, much human misery has been contained (where it can be afforded). Genetic modification probably offers the great leap forward in human health for the future even though it is clouded with moral uncertainties and the dark shadows of Nazi experiments before World War II. The principle is already in wide use in plant propagation, agricultural pest control and animal breeding. Human experiments in a range of important areas are taking place and producing some startling results.

Perhaps we'll even locate a gene for susceptibility to the common cold, though the work of Andrewes and his heirs makes that seem a ridiculous proposition. We will certainly have a new armoury to tackle organic conditions such as hypertension (high blood pressure) leading to stroke, heart disease and cancer – the major killers in the developed world today.

CHAPTER 6

HOW DIET, SUNSHINE & ACTIVITY INTERACT

Dr Zane Kime, in *Sunlight Could Save Your Life* (1980), put his head on the block with a firm assertion: 'if developing the immune response of the individual assumes its proper emphasis in medical thinking, sunlight's contribution to that goal would be recognised.' Though this view, in the present 'politically correct' but incorrect circumstances, may be sacrilegious by running against the popular tide, it cannot be avoided as a central point of focus in the saga of the common cold.

Kime again: 'the sun continues to be the potent, life-giving, health-dealing force for modern man that it was instinctively recognised to be by primitive man ... separation from sunlight will result in disease just as surely as will separation from fresh air, food and/or water'.

Then he makes one other observation that is vital to the case to be made out later: 'It is important to note that cholesterol and vitamin D are related for, when cholesterol in the skin is exposed to sunlight, it may easily be changed to vitamin D and thereby be made harmless to the body.'

We should go further. It would be made beneficial to the body and is one of the processes whereby sunlight is so essential, but only one. Drugs prescribed to eliminate excessive levels of 'bad' cholesterol, by this yardstick, could cause some serious problems.

The *Israeli Journal of Medicine* (April 1995) points out that the synthesis of vitamin D is dependent on UVB frequency light reaching the lower epidermal (skin) layers. Vitamin D levels are significantly higher in whites compared with blacks who, nevertheless have a higher bone mass (no doubt because of some other supplementary or complementary process, or genetic traits).

In 1985, in a ground breaking study, Professor M. J. Lillyquist, professor of psychology at Wisconsin University, set out in *Sunlight and Health* to reveal the idiocy of the present attitudes to sun exposure. In an opening summary of the sun's redeeming features, he listed:

- Vitamin D synthesis is increased.
- By inducing pigmentation, tanning, it protects the skin from the potentially harmful effects of over-exposure.
- Lowers blood pressure and reduces harmful cholesterol.
- On entering the eyes, triggers internal reactions that affect blood, bones, protein levels, and glands and organs.
- Increases resistance to disease and even cures some conditions.

This is hardly an extreme position and some strong support for Lillyquist's views will be offered as we proceed.

Without sunlight, the source and energiser of all life on earth, we lose muscle tone, become weak, sexually apathetic and depressed. Sunlight, therefore, is necessary for normal human functioning. Christopher Hufeland knew this in 1897 after observing people who had been kept in dungeons. Adequate exposure to sunlight is basic to health. An old German proverb says the funeral coach turns twice as often on the shady side of the street.

Lillyquist introduces another important principle.

'In maintaining health, we are our own physicians for we are the ones best suited to guide our actions, our habits, and our lives... Balance and moderation are the secrets of good health.'

This applies as much to using the resources of sunlight as to anything else. It was known by 1877 that sunlight killed bacteria and that short invisible UV waves had the greatest antibacterial effect. A Dane, Niels Finsen, was awarded a Nobel Prize in 1903 for discovering the use of artificially produced UV light to cure TB of the skin, Lupus vulgaris. The results were 'almost magical'.

Other discoveries were made. Patients treated with UV radiation every five days showed an 8-10 per cent fall in blood pressure – and the effects lasted for months. (Is this why primitive peoples living in tribal conditions do not show rises of blood pressure with increasing age?) Having observed the curing of meat with sunlight, the idea was tested on war wounds. One almost hopeless victim showed a significant improvement after less than two hours and the wound healed normally.

Synthesis of vitamin D through the skin facilitates the absorption of calcium by the gut and prevents rickets, a bone deficiency condition. The early Egyptians recorded this fact and the principle was used to good effect in sun-deprived northern England in the first half of the century when living and working conditions deprived many people of sufficient light. Sunlight was also used to cure TB and a range of skin disorders.

There followed the science of heliotherapy in which sunlight was even promoted as an antidote to old age. Solar therapy was widely used to treat the wounded of World War I. Americans, Lillyquist reports, were often exhorted to site their homes at 45 degrees to the north/south axis so all the walls of the house received sun at some point in the year. Cities, at this time, were regarded by many people as 'havens of disease', so much so that 'sunlight cities' were planned in the US, no doubt to the undying benefit of their citizens.

The 'healthy tan' became fashionable and no good film hero would be photographed without one, along with a cigarette, of course. Pallid skin was equated with ill health and a suntan became a status symbol (after the car). The whole idea was, like the present condemnation of the sun's effects, taken to ridiculous extremes. Here note the earlier comments about 'balance'.

By 1920, a link between sunlight and skin cancers was known among physicians. Certain forms of plant oils or perfume additives were known to cause dermatitis, too. Then it was discovered that the sun had the potential to damage the retina of the eye. Sunlight was already becoming in the eyes of many medicos a malefactor. Viewers of the BBC production, *The World at War*, may have observed General Rommel's melanoma, which prompted his return to Germany at a critical point in the North African campaign. In later footage, he returned to the North African theatre of war and was apparently cured with no obvious scarring, so German doctors must have known how to handle the problem.

Then came sunglasses.

After long years of sun worship, a response that was slow to be discredited in the sun-deprived northern climes of Europe where the annual pilgrimage to the sun was pursued with an ardour in which no affordable expense was spared, there was in the US a sharp reaction and the need to cover up again. The hat and sunscreen and long sleeves became *de rigeur* for the cautious who feared skin cancers, though the topless belles of the beach were motivated by more primeval urges.

'Now,' says Lillyquist (and you'll recall he was arguing this 10 years ago), 'we must re-evaluate the effects of sunlight – and not just as a new found aphrodisiac.' (He was referring to an article that had appeared in 1981 in the US magazine *Harper's Bazaar* in which sunbathing was accorded a key role in maintaining sexual potency and desire.)

In some senses the cancer scare was to go full circle because it was discovered that exposure to sunlight could prevent cancers in other parts of the body. Dr Sigmund Peller, of the John Hopkins School of Hygiene, had gathered evidence as early as 1940 suggesting that getting sufficient sunlight to cause a (curable) skin cancer could well be a reasonable price to pay for a significantly lower incidence of more serious cancers. Now, of course, we know that careful exposure to sunlight behind a gradually built protective suntan can offer the benefits without the risks.

'The sun', Lillyquist says, 'is down but not out. Until the early 1980s, it appeared evident that sunlight was going the way of cigarettes and illicit drugs – each was declared harmful, and the most sensible strategy for health educators was to inform and dissuade the public from their use.'

But the burial of sunlight was premature.

Lillyquist picks up on a report in the August 1982 issue of *The Lancet* in which it is claimed that workers in offices lit by fluorescent tubes appeared more at risk of melanomas than those working outdoors. While it is unlikely that such a statement would be true for countries with hot sunny climates, it poses the question of whether these cancers were a consequence of lack of sunlight on the workers' bodies or some problem inherent in the limited spectrum of fluorescent light.

Perhaps the most interesting claim was that indoor workers with melanomas tended to develop the cancer on a part of the body not normally exposed to the sun.

Then there is the equally intriguing matter of melatonin production. This hormone is secreted and circulated in the hours of darkness and production is 'switched off' by bright light. If there is insufficient exposure to light to stop melatonin production, the inevitable consequence is depression and sickness despite the fact that melatonin is essential to a functional immune system. Scientists working in the Arctic in the dark winter period reported a decline in sex drive and potency, insomnia, weakness, hair loss, depression, and irritability. However, it was thought that lack of sunlight was only part of the story. Eskimos suffer high rates of TB, rheumatic fever, hepatitis, diabetes, leukemia, cardiovascular disease (despite their fish oil diet) and dental caries. Suicide and alcoholism is rife, too. Again, sunlight deprivation is not the whole story.

The prevalence of colds among coal miners who work underground is well known and a continuing problem. But is there a seasonal pattern? We need more research on many of these claims.

Is this simply a matter of a vitamin D shortfall, in part replaced in the salted fish diet of many North Europeans? Herrings are rich in vitamin D and the salt ensured safe storage for the winter months when bad weather could restrict fishing. Vitamin D, a hormone produced by the action of sun on the skin, enables the bones to absorb calcium. Even where there are adequate levels of calcium in the diet, it will not be absorbed unless vitamin D is present. Lillyquist refers to an American study in which a group of elderly men were deprived of sunlight for seven weeks. By the end of the trial their calcium absorption had fallen by 60 per cent.

Even on this scanty evidence, the sun has to be seen as a benefactor, though one that demands respect. The problem with maximising the good effects is really down to the manner in which people use sunlight to advantage rather than their detriment.

In principle it is only the fair skinned, or those people who have never exposed their bodies to light since childhood, or ever, who do not develop their own sunscreen of pigment. Once that pigment has been activated, it comes back quickly whenever the once suntanned person is again exposed. The secret of the successful sunbather is never to get sunburnt. That means careful and thoughtful exposure rather than lashings of questionable chemicals which may, or may not, provide some protection. A few heavily promoted products have been shown to be surprisingly ineffective.

Even occasional sunburn, Lillyquist argues, does not seem to do much harm to the skin though many skin specialists would disagree with this claim. He admits, however, that fair skinned people with blue eyes who redden rather than tan should be particularly cautious in direct sun.

Why, then, does Australia lead the melanoma league?

Lillyquist believes this is because a high proportion of residents are descendants of Anglo-Saxons with little pigment and a poor adaptation to that environment. There is probably a complex of interlocking reasons, not least that Australians have been exposed directly to doses of nuclear radiation. Not only were 'dirty' nuclear weapons tested in the middle of the land mass at Maralinga, but they were tested repeatedly offshore at Bikini Atoll and off Western Australia. Until recently, the French were still testing at Mururoa Atoll. That's not to say radioactive fallout, some of which fell on cities, directly causes melanomas, but exposure to some forms of radiation is known to affect the body's immune system. An inhibited immune system is more likely to fail to remove cancerous cells.

Cancer cells appear in all humans but the immune system seems to handle this problem for most people at least until old age. If, however, *over exposure* to sunlight, and the consequent high levels of radiation, acts to depress the function of the immune system, the problem may be explained that way. In the case of fluorescent lighting, Lillyquist claims there is evidence that suntanned people working under fluorescent lights appear to be better protected against ill effects because of the melanin levels in their skins. Consider another possibility. Some drugs in common use such as the antibiotic tetracycline, many high blood pressure medications, and some antidepressants increase the photosensitivity of the skin. Users should ask their physicians to state whether a prescribed drug is likely to increase sun sensitivity, particularly when they have a vulnerable skin type. Many over the counter medications can cause similar effects.

Sunlight on a bright day is about 100,000 lux compared with artificial light which generally ranges up to 3,000 lux maximum. We know that exposure to light for excessive periods can disrupt the serotonin/melatonin cycles, and accelerate growth and sexual maturation. For example, the testes of drakes exposed to red light for long periods may increase in size by up to 16 times and this could presage a significant increase in the output of the male hormone testosterone.

Perhaps this was the origin of the 'red light' district.

Bright light stimulates the production of cortisol, an activating hormone, but excessive production causes fatigue after a while. A researcher who exposed a test subject to fluorescent light for two weeks recorded rising levels of the hormones ACTH and cortisol, too. Both these chemicals are often described as 'stress hormones'.

If the eyes are the entry point of light and the source of its effects, do sunglasses protect the eyes adequately or inhibit other necessary functions? Lillyquist cites a test case where the UV passed by the lens was double the level that would have been received by the user if no sunglasses had been worn!

A 12-year study of 4,000 male students at Cornell University tracked a direct relationship between climatic factors such as temperature and hours of sunshine with the frequency of colds. When chronic cold sufferers were given 10 minutes a week exposure to ultraviolet light, there was a negligible effect. When the exposure was increased to 30 minutes, the number of colds was almost halved. The Russians, too, used UV lamps in factories hit by a high incidence of colds among workers to reduce the number of colds by half.

Don't be tempted at this point to put colds down simply to UV exposure. There is much more to the story than that.

Jacob Liberman, in *Light – The Medicine of the Future* (1991) takes us a step further. He has pioneered the therapeutic use of light and colour and what is termed 'the art of mind/body integration'. In a country where the constitution protects the right of free speech, the extent of loose speech is phenomenal and the West Coast in particular seems to produce more cranks to the square metre than elsewhere in the world. Don't be tempted to include Liberman in this motley collection even if his language at times suggests a radical perspective.

In the foreword to Liberman's book, Dr John Ott, who specialises in the relatively new field of photobiology, refutes any idea that sunlight is detrimental to health. He, too, blames this false consciousness on financial and commercial interests and effective propaganda.

'Vitamins,' he argues, 'will not solve the problems caused by a lack of the appropriate wavelengths of light necessary to create complete metabolism. There is no question in my mind that the visible portion of the spectrum, as well as a certain point beyond, especially the UV, act as the ignition system for all human biological functions.'

That's quite a leap from the simplistic idea that it's all down to sunshine and vitamin D, but it makes a lot of sense when applied to the wide range of clearly related ideas considered so far. Liberman sees the body as a kind of living photo-cell regulated by light entering through the eyes. (Why only the eyes? Perhaps because the writer is an eye specialist. What about the light sensitivity of the skin and other organs?) Light becomes in his view a nutrient which catalyses biological combustion in humans just as photosynthesis takes place in plants. Any plant, or human for that matter, deprived of light dies when the stored resources are spent.

'Modern technological advancements, such as most fluorescent lights, sunglasses, tanning lotions and our general indoor lifestyles, may in fact be harming us more than helping us', he says. 'Far from being hazardous, UV is one of the most biologically active and important portions of the electromagnetic spectrum.' No mention here of the hole in the ozone layer, the oft-stated reason for 'covering up'.

He makes the critical point that all the energy we take into our bodies is derived from the sun. The sun's energy, through photosynthesis, is stored in plants which are then eaten by animals and humans. Digestion is essentially a process of breaking down, transferring and utilising this light created energy. In 1979, Martinek and Berezin hypothesised that light and colour played 'a remarkable role' in how effectively certain enzyme systems regulated biological activity within the body.

Liberman goes further.

Light, he says, is not only about seeing, about vision, but for acting on the hypothalamus. One part of this organ controls the sympathetic nervous system and stimulates hormone production. The other controls the secretions of the pituitary gland, thereby significantly affecting the endocrine system which regulates metabolism. (Is this why the Anglo-Saxon pioneers in Australia, particularly farmers, developed big noses and extremities with elongated forearms, and their offspring gained significantly in height?)

The pineal gland, or what was once known as the third eye and about which there is now a considerable body of research to be found in any university library, now comes into the story. This gland is only the size of a pea in most humans but it acts as a sort of light meter, receiving light activated information from the eyes through the hypothalamus and in turn sending out hormonal 'messages' to other parts of the brain and body. This may involve the length of daylight, so it is 'season sensitive'. It co-ordinates the relationship between an individual organism and its environment.

Now the pineal, among many functions, controls the release of the hormone melatonin – the direct source of most of the discomforts of jetlag. Some years ago in Australia, a researcher found that melatonin levels – the hormone is usually released between 2am and 3am at maximum levels – could adjust in response to quite small volumes of light provided exposure lasted for an hour or more.

More than 100 body functions have daily rhythms which are regulated by light. If light is not perceived, there is a significant disturbance in physical and emotional stability. Liberman believes that different colours (wavelengths of light or radiations) interact in various ways with the endocrine system to stimulate or inhibit hormone production. (Remember those drakes?) At the University of Freiberg in Germany, it was shown that the wrong kind of light can cripple a plant while normal light exposure allows it to grow normally. Most owners of potted plants, particularly those ailing in artificially lit hallways or offices, will understand that.

The vitamin D manufactured in the body as a hormone and derived from the antecedent cholesterol is cholecalciferol and it occurs in direct response to UV exposure. It is quite different from the commercially produced vitamin D3 found in most dairy foods, while the ergocalciferol found in vitamin D tablets and fortified foods is different again. The natural vitamin D3 is never toxic whereas the artificial D2 taken in excess can be toxic. So, when we talk about vitamin substitutes, we are not necessarily dealing with the same chemicals or an identical metabolic process. Neither are we adequately accounting for photosynthesis. It is not too hard to see now why susceptibility to illness should increase in the winter months. Lower levels of light intensity and shorter days, not to mention the cold that forces people indoors unless they take to the ski slopes or travel to sunnier climes for holidays, acts in much the same way that sun deprivation affects Arctic scientists or coal miners.

Waiting in the background, in an uneasy truce with the immune system, lie the viral predators – not, of course, that all viral agents are harmful. Roughly half of all viruses recovered from their human hosts have failed to produce an active illness, or at least we are not today aware of any malevolence so they may have another symbiotic role to play.

When the effects of sun deprivation are linked with other predisposing factors, and the malfunction or inhibition of the immune system, a much more vulnerable situation is created.

Earlier we mentioned the impact of excessive physical training. A recent study of 60 road runners, nine women and 51 men, demonstrated that the incidence of upper respiratory infections increased with the number of road miles run each year. High levels of training became 'a significant risk factor'. Over-training creates a complex health syndrome of which impairment of the immune system is but one component. The interaction of the nervous and immune systems, through the hypothalamus-pituitary-adrenal axis, exerts profound effects on the athletes' susceptibility to disease. Yet these people can't do their training anywhere except out of doors so they are being exposed to daylight for reasonable periods of time unless they train exclusively after work and at night (which could be the case).

Conversely, lack of exercise and a gradually declining metabolic rate will also predispose people to rising levels of infection, as well as obesity and muscle wastage. Even three gentle walks a week for 30 minutes or so will keep the incidence of illness down, especially if you walk in sunlight. One key to health, and preventing overweight which may also be a negative factor for a strong immune system, is to balance dietary 'inputs and outputs'. The slimming industry is a multi-billion rip-off around the world. Millions of enthusiastic people diet aggressively and reduce weight for relatively short periods, often damaging their health and immunity in the process, without realising that one will only put on weight if the food intake is not metabolised adequately and expended. That's too complex a process to detail here.

Then remember the mental or psychological aspect.

Australian studies have shown that the death rate among those recently bereaved is three to 12 times higher than otherwise. In Britain, among 4,486 widowers aged 54 and older, death rates were 40 per cent higher in the first six months of bereavement. Other factors may be at work here, of course – poor personal care and diet, failure to take medications, ignoring the need for medical help – which would all increase the death risk.

Even drug 'misuse' could play a part.

According to the *American Family Physician* (April 1995), sore throat is the most common ailment presenting to physicians. An Australian study of 284 physicians examined the inappropriate use of antibiotic prescriptions for this condition. The participants were given four medical scenarios and asked to specify what action they would take. The results showed 97 per cent would prescribe an antibiotic for a child with tonsillitis and 10 per cent would do the same for an adult with a likely *viral* infection. Of the sample, 70 per cent said they would prescribe an antibiotic for an adult presenting with glandular fever (infectious mononucleosis) and nearly one third would prescribe an antibiotic for a child with what appeared to be a viral sore throat.

The main first choice of antibiotic was penicillin (71 per cent) with erythromycin as the first choice of fewer than 4 per cent of those questioned. However, this drug was the main second choice of 83 per cent. Then comes the disturbing aspect. In one fifth, 20 per cent, of cases, the first choice of antibiotic was an inappropriate broad spectrum agent. (First reported in the *British Journal of General Practice*, November 1994).

Add to this worrying study, for example, the poor prescription standards of some general practitioners in areas such as heart disease, high blood pressure and arthritis, where many of the drugs in common use are known to impact on the functioning of the immune system to an unknown extent. The incidence of colds may again be affected by other forms of treatment such as the unnecessary use of X-rays. How many patients were warned of the possible outcomes?

There is current interest in the use of a zinc supplement in lozenge form to combat rhinovirus infections and treat a cold after onset. This, of course, is not the purpose in this book which is to stop colds altogether by boosting immunity. The results of a clinical trial published recently in *Annals of Internal Medicine*, while suggesting there may be treatment benefits, do not really advance the cause significantly. Microbiologist Dr Geoffrey Scott, of University College London Hospital, is sceptical. He was quoted in *The Independent* (18 June 1996) as saying: 'Once you have a cold, you've got a cold. You have to ask whether it's worthwhile shortening its length. Whether it's necessary from a medical point of view is very dubious.

Finally, we have the crimes of the cook. Cooking changes the structure of many foods and affects the manner in which they are digested and metabolised. It may also reduce or change the vitamin content and render otherwise valuable chemicals inaccessible to the human body. Diet clearly is important and intelligent supplementation must play a part in the context of light exposure and body chemistry we have considered so far.

In many ways, civilisation is the culprit.

Yet, despite all these shortcomings – light deprivation, cooked and highly processed foods, clothing and indoor living, the stresses of the workplace and lifestyle, longevity in the developed industrial nations is now much higher than it was a century ago so we must be getting some of it right. Unfortunately, we are still getting too many colds – and that is what concerns us here.

CHAPTER 7

EFFECTS OF AN INDUSTRIAL LIFESTYLE

Let's restate the problem in a different way. Why is it that so few people, relatively, succumb to a pathogen when exposed? Those committed to a psychological perspective on medicine like to talk of 'resistance resources'. Researchers at Boston University's School of Medicine speculated that people succumb to illness and seek medical help when they perceive a distressing life situation which cannot be resolved effectively. This results in a sense of helplessness and negative emotions which erodes resistance to disease and makes them more vulnerable to the ever-present pathogens.

Beliefs, in this view, affect health.

Medical research is replete with examples and studies which show individuals carrying a virus but not developing the disease it causes. For Blair Justice (see page 61), this reflects attitudes of pessimism or optimism. In the light of what has gone before, we would want to be more pragmatic and give the immune system a key role. The mental aspects of disease come into play at this level as a *chemical response* to emotional perceptions.

One of the traps for researchers so far has been the western way of 'doing science' based on the philosophy, or way of thinking, of logical positivism which rests on the idea of cause and effect, stimulus and response. Once you move to multicausal explanations or to relating phenomena like sickness and circumstances, you remove many of the blocks to understanding illness, and in particular the common cold.

When bugs were seen to 'cause' disease, medical practice focused on the need to control the spread of bacilli, viruses, funguses and all the other pathogens that were seen as the infecting agents.

We developed ideas like 'smoking causes lung cancer'. Apart from the fact that many heavy smokers did not develop lung cancer, even though they may have suffered from other life threatening conditions that were directly attributable to cigarette smoking, this left much to be desired as a coherent all embracing explanation of lung cancer. Many people who have never smoked also get this disease.

No one to my knowledge has proposed that poorly shielded X-ray equipment could just as easily have been responsible for many of the lung cancers.

What about the 98 per cent of Caucasian Americans who do not succumb to the endemic TB bacillus? Or those people in the polio epidemics after World War II who carried the virus but only suffered a mild form of the disease? Or the so-called Asian flu which ravaged western populations in the late 1960s or early 1970s when there were no antibodies to the virus in affected populations? Only some people succumbed and subsequent research shows that those with low morale suffered more debilitating symptoms and slower recovery rates.

Likewise AIDS. A retrovirus, HIV, predisposes a carrier to succumb to the syndrome in which the immune system attacks itself and creates susceptibility to other forms of illness but does not itself *cause* the fatal illness. It undermines the body's ability to defend itself from attack. You could be one of the millions of people who are HIV positive and, like many who are TB positive, remain healthy in much the same way that hepatitis B carriers do not necessarily succumb to the disease.

Cause and effect is not a good way to explain illness.

Germ theory, useful in its time to enable research and as a simple way of looking at disease, now has significant shortcomings. We have to explain phenomena that defy such approaches. Why, for example, do certain pathogens 'cause' different diseases in different people?

At the end stage, it may be better to say that personal wellbeing is shaped more by the way we perceive the quality of our lives and intimate relationships and our ability to cope with life rather than mere germs. However, we have to take into account that industrial society offers a troublesome environment for an organism that evolved in a vastly different set of environmental conditions.

Few medical researchers working in the area would now dispute the idea that stress and disease are funtionally related. Once you accept that proposition, you are admitting that there is a mental perspective to illness, or rather a close relationship between what happens in the mind and to the body. Quite apart from the tensions and inconsistencies of working with other people, there are direct physical stresses that have to be taken into account in understanding the common cold.

That does not mean that colds are 'just psychological'. We have already seen that this is not the case.

In an earlier chapter we saw that coal miners working underground traditionally have been very susceptible to repeated colds, apparently as a result of sunlight deprivation. In the modern industrial world many people work unusual hours in difficult circumstances – hospital staff, aircrew, cab drivers, police and security guards, service station attendants in 24-hour outlets, and all the rest. These people have to adapt to different circumstances. Provided they always live according to a consistent routine, they can make that adaptation successfully and compensate for lost sunlight exposure by taking their recreation at different times of day.

Nevertheless, there is a lot of evidence to suggest that shift workers suffer much more physical stress and higher rates of illness than the majority of day workers. If they work only for periods on night shift then revert to day work, the problems are compounded.

Even day workers have problems.

Apart from the narrow spectrum fluorescent lights discussed

earlier, they may spend long hours staring at visual display terminal screens, whether or not the microwaves and electromagnetic fields generated are harmful. They may breathe an exotic array of pollutants from photocopiers and other electronic equipment. They are fed processed air through an air-conditioning system that could well be dispensing a sub-standard product. Not only that, the conditioned air may be excessively hot or cold, humid or dry, and it could even disperse a range of bacterial agents the like of which produce Legionnaire's disease. Some may be working in sick buildings.

These people travel to and from work in public transport that may leave a lot to be desired in terms of comfort or cleanliness. Or they crawl and jostle to work in traffic congestion that leaves their lungs assailed by diesel fumes, carbon monoxide and a host of other pollutants or irritants.

When they finally get home at night after all these attacks on the integrity of the immune system, they may heat their homes excessively, spray insecticides too generously to dispose of household or garden pests, use too many hazardous cleaning agents, and finally curl up in front of the telly for the evening with a prepacked meal of dubious nutritional value. Or, worse, a beer and a home delivered pizza.

All in all this is not a good scenario for healthy living – or more particularly to keep the immune system functioning at peak.

Quite apart from the stresses these lifestyle factors impose on a person physically, there are the relationship and parental stresses superimposed on top. Here we move into a difficult area because we do not have many solid facts on the way in which the immune system handles emotional problems. Or even whether substances that we consider pollutant may not also have some beneficial effects.

The faster pace of life of the city may even increase resistance to disease because city dwellers develop a more vigorous metabolism. Certainly, one observes that the majority of people in most cities seem healthy enough and have adapted to their apparently 'unnatural' circumstances. The stimulation provided by broad social contacts and the wider exposure to pathogens could be beneficial by sensitising the immune system to a broader range of viral, bacterial and other assailants.

Let's not rush to the easy conclusion that urban life is 'unnatural' and therefore bad. It may in practice be a much better way to organise human needs socially, economically and politically. What concerns us here is how we adapt to these circumstances in a *healthy* way so we do not constantly get colds, or other annoying and uncomfortable upper respiratory infections.

To do this, we have to accept the urban and industrial lifestyle and fit our protective regime into that mould.

The key, then, is to identify the factors that will sustain, or hopefully enhance, the functioning of the immune system and maximise this potential once we know why people get colds repeatedly. In the final chapter, we'll run out a strategy for long term cold prevention. Here we must separate out those aspects of modern life which are **not** relevant so they don't clutter up our understanding of those that are.

We have already established (1) that you do not catch cold by getting cold/wet/chilled or coming home shivering from a football match. You succumb to a cold or similar upper respiratory infection because your immune system fails to detect an antigen, or is in some way inhibited from functioning effectively.

Because the pathogens responsible for the cold are ever present, there is little point (2) in approaching external sources of infection in a paranoid fashion and going out of your way to avoid carriers and cross-infection. Provided your immune system has been previously exposed to that virus, you have little to fear. Indeed, you may have something to gain by keeping your immune system on red alert.

Denial of sunlight (3) is clearly a constant problem that, if sustained, inevitably produces rising levels of disease though we have a problem with the Spitzbergen study. These people did not succumb to colds until, as the weather warmed, a visiting supply ship was thought to have brought a new source of bugs. If the viral agents are ever present, why did the scientists not have colds all the winter? (Probably because of the very low temperatures which, in effect, put the bugs 'on ice' until the thaw began.)

Observation suggests (4) that the danger periods for colds are the warmer autumn and spring periods, not the deep midwinter when snow lies on the ground. That fits with the point above and with experience. Flu epidemics, however, have their own dynamic and may not entirely fit this pattern because they concern another kind of virus with an ability to multiply and spread worldwide in certain environmental conditions. Whether or not there is any mileage in the idea of external factors like sunspot activity, and we should treat ideas like this with some caution, there are certainly circumstances that enable a new flu virus to wreak havoc among people who have not been exposed before.

Here we are dealing with the common cold, permanently if all goes well, not flu epidemics. We need (5) to separate the two illnesses in our minds and keep them apart in terms of prevention. *The immune system has to encounter a particular form of a virus to memorise its characteristics and recognise it again.* Even then, because of the ready mutations of some viruses, minor changes in gene structure may make that particular antigen unrecognisable.

We are concerned only with the 200 or more viruses and commonly encountered bacterial agents that cause most of our ills.

The economic realities of most people's lives are that they have to do many things they would, in an ideal world, prefer not to do – commuting, working in crowded uncomfortable conditions, racing to and from the local school to deliver and collect children, overtime or working excessive hours, putting up with demanding and unreasonable superiors. These things we cannot change just to avoid getting colds. What we have to do (6) is adapt our bodies to the demands we are compelled to make on them so we stay healthy.

However much we feel threatened (7) by pollutants, nuclear weapon testing, processed and junk foods, drugs, rising levels of violent crime or even mindless television, there is nothing much we can do to change these things except switch off or go away to live on a Pacific Island. Even then some militaristic world power may be there to radioactivate bits of it. The negative aspects of contemporary life have to be taken as given and the immune system must learn to cope.

People, inevitably, will be assailed constantly by media pundits to eat this or not eat that, to jog or meditate, or to avoid stress and tribulation by various psychological means. This propaganda, too, often clouds the real issues and serves commercial or even political interests, or the promotional needs of the media because fear sells as many newspapers or magazines as sex or the indiscretions of the Royal Family. Anyone who wants to protect their health (8) must start by trying to get their mind straight and evaluating all this puff and nonsense sensibly in the light of personal observation and experience.

Adopt a sceptical standpoint.

Lastly, for all the stresses of today's urban world, people live longer, have greater freedom from disease, and enjoy a much more adequate and comfortable lifestyle. Even the much berated supermarket distributes fresh food cheaply, efficiently and hygienically. What really matters (9) is how you perceive your place in this world, positively or negatively. Even if you are unfortunate enough to be one of the rising numbers of people displaced by technology and thus unemployed, there are still some big pluses in life that can be turned to good health advantage.

A very old friend of mine in his 90s, one evening by the fire a long time ago, described in detail his memories of life in London at the end of the 19th century. It quickly became clear that neither of us would for a moment want to return to that lifestyle of social injustice, street hazards and economic uncertainty. In 1945, Andrewes had only a sketchy view of the common cold and the elusive virus thought to be responsible. We have come a long way in 100 years and a lot of what has happened, excluding warfare, has been for the good.

Now, if we can only rid ourselves of the common cold...

CHAPTER 8

NEVER HAVE ANOTHER COLD

This is no idle or sensational claim. We can't promise you escape from a new flu virus which your immune system hasn't met before, but within reason you should be able – if you follow the suggestions below – to rid yourself and your family of colds. Young children, especially when they start in a creche, or kindergarten, or at school, will inevitably encounter many new pathogens. Depending on their overall health (and how many antibiotics have been poured down their throats), they will succumb to some of these to develop a fully armed immune system. Once this is done they, like the adult members of the family, should be equally immune to most cold viruses.

A word of caution. High fevers in very young children with a developing immune system can be dangerous and require treatment. One consequence of a high fever can be convulsions, and a parent encountering this for the first time may be alarmed. Seek professional help if this occurs.

Let's return for the moment to the work of Professor Dwyer. He says: 'The discovery that a normal part of the immune response to infection produces some of the major *symptoms* of infection rapidly led to further work. This has demonstrated convincingly that, when we feel ill because of an infection, it is because our bodies are caught up as innocent bystanders in a fight to the death being waged by lymphocytes and their partners and the invaders they are trying to eliminate.'

The majority of micro-organisms that attack us, however, don't produce any toxins so it is our response, the immune process, that produces the symptoms we interpret as 'illness'.

Dwyer stresses that fatigue is a protective response which warns one not to overdo it. 'The immune system has learnt to trigger the receptor in our brain that declares fatigue so that, when we're infected, we rest, and this enhances our immune system's capacity to fight infection.'

In other words, the body seeks to regulate the output and distribution of energy and healing resources. Hence the long standing medical advice to treat a cold by going to bed and drinking lemon and honey. There is, however, another school of thought. If, when assailed by relatively minor infections, you boost your metabolic rate like the man referred to earlier who went out and started digging vigorously in the garden, the 'hyped up' metabolism gives the immune system a helpful kick along. You may also recall that part of this man's stated aim was 'to work up a sweat' hence lift body temperature – and that may be where most of the beneficial effect lay, at least in his experience.

Dwyer makes a number of other important observations:

- Severe depression, for example bereavement, can affect T-cell function and therefore compromise the immune system
- T-cell production, and the natural cut-off point in human life that results from expending the stock of immune system cells, is 'markedly delayed' in the underfed. We don't know why, or what the benefit to the organism might be.
- Zinc and magnesium are essential for normal immune function.
- Vitamin deficiencies restrict immune function, the vitamins A and C in particular. Likewise a lack of iron, folic acid, zinc, riboflavin, or niacin. That said, there is no evidence that taking excessive amounts of any of these food additives in any way increases immunity. They have only to be present in sufficient amounts for the body to function normally.
- Perhaps 80 per cent of all human disease could be ended with our mastery of the immune response.

- Mind rules the body and, in particular, mind and the immune system 'talk' to each other constantly.
- Hormones are the products of the endocrine system which, when released, act to make us do something different.
- Some individuals may enhance the efficiency of their immune systems under stress, perhaps because they respond positively. In others, who approach their situation negatively, immunity may be inhibited.
- The mind/immune system link runs both ways so it is likely that a person with a 'strong' or effective immune system is also better able to cope.
- Stress in most people causes the brain to initiate a series of chemical responses that helps to alleviate the stress when the action works. Coping, in other words. Where the chemical response does not alleviate the stress, some immune responses may be 'shut down' and this may result in disease.
- A person's ability to cope with a stressful event will determine whether the immune system performs as it should.
- Researchers found that the secretion of a natural immunoglobulin to boost immunity, in this case a substance that protects the mucous membranes of the upper airways, was suppressed in students under stress during exams. As a consequence, *they were more susceptible to infections of the upper respiratory tract.*

The common cold is a problem because we are culturally conditioned to expect to catch colds from others, that the illness is 'trivial' and therefore not worth protecting ourselves against in any concerted way, and that in some senses a cold is as good as a rest. In part, community attitudes towards the common cold derive from the Anglo-Saxon perception that the cold is inherently a response to a relatively warm, wet and often depressing climate. Other nationalities have medical 'obsessions' like the French concern with their livers (given the level of alcohol consumption, particularly with black coffee for breakfast, this is not surprising).

Part of this 'cold culture' is the treatment adopted as a matter of course when a child succumbs.

As we saw earlier, most of the present treatments are 'good' for a cold only in the sense that they prolong the illness, inhibit immune response, and predispose the sufferer to repeat the process several times during the winter. We are taught in childhood that:

1. Everyone gets colds.
2. The symptoms are 'the illness' not the signs of an immune response.
3. The symptoms must be treated to make the cold better and that freedom from symptoms indicates healing is taking place, or has already finished.
4. Certain specific symptoms such as a runny nose are an indispensable part of having a cold and unavoidable.
5. Everyone gets colds 'all the time', that is regularly – and there is nothing to be considered abnormal in that.
6. You 'catch' cold because of some external occurrence – exposure to sources of infection, because you are 'run down', infected by the workplace air conditioning system, or you have been 'overdoing it'.
7. Other members of your family or work associates will 'catch your cold' if they're not exceptionally lucky.
8. Children bring home all sorts of nasty bugs from school and 'infect' the rest of the family.

This cold culture lulls people into a false security. Because of the myths and conventional wisdom, they fail to see the need to protect themselves from this constant viral assault and, instead, just go to bed with the lemon and honey. This has reduced the pressure to find a cure for colds, or more accurately, to *prevent* colds. Most people, even today, would imagine that you could only end the scourge of the cold by eliminating all the causal viruses with the other pathogens that produce similar symptoms.

To prevent colds, then, requires a change of attitude.

Succumbing to the common cold is neither necessary nor inevitable. It happens because we fail to protect ourselves by maintaining an efficient immune system against all odds. Given the extraordinary range of antigens responsible for colds, there is no hope of creating resistance to each one by overcoming infection and developing the necessary antibodies. Assuming there are only 200 viruses implicated, and we will certainly discover more before we've finished, that a cold takes on average a week to overcome, and you were somehow exposed to all these viruses, you would be facing in a lifetime around 1400 days or almost four years of constant illness.

That, of course, is a farcical idea.

The alternative is to build effective resistance and sustain the immune system much as you would the family car – constant maintenance, sufficient fuel and oil, and new tyres and battery when necessary. It also needs washing down regularly and some polish to defend it from sun, salt or water. When something serious goes wrong, it is probably because you failed to maintain the vehicle adequately or were exposed to an unusual and unrecognised hazard. And when the vehicle is old, it becomes much more susceptible to mechanical failure.

Without pressing this analogy too far, it's clear that effective maintenance has to start from Day One.

Physical fitness, to a normal and comfortable standard of activity and muscle development, has to start in early childhood. Few children will fail to get enough exercise but some, for various reasons, may be deprived of fresh air, outdoor activity and sunshine. People who live in warm climates near the sea have all the resources of physical fitness on hand, but those who live in congested and polluted cities, without garden or recreation space, have many more problems.

Some parents go to extremes, 'pushing' their children to excel in sports by pursuing an unnecessary, and demonstrably unhealthy, intensity of physical training. We have seen earlier that this can undermine the immune response, particularly at adolescence when profound hormonal changes are taking place. Simultaneously, we impose on adolescents heavy school performance demands which, as stressors, link with excessive physical stresses to depress immunity.

A happy child will be a healthy child even though there may be occasional brushes with viral infections to which it must create immunity unless inherited. If a child is tired, he or she should rest. If a child is constantly tired and 'run down', there is something wrong with metabolic function. If a child succumbs constantly to one infection after another, the immune system is not up to par and a change of lifestyle is clearly needed.

Once the physical resources of the child have been developed to a point of 'fitness', that foundation will last for life. Physical fitness is not about being superior to others in some athletic pursuit, it's about coping with the demands of everyday life while remaining healthy and energetic.

That doesn't mean that a young adult can opt out of maintaining physical fitness during life. But with reasonable exercise and recreation, the physical capacities developed in childhood, along with the stock of T-cells, should sustain health and promote a reasonable span of life. So what goes wrong?

Any number of life threatening events can disrupt the normal course of healthy life and by so doing undermine or burn up the resources of the immune system. A serious illness, to which neither parent nor child had previously been exposed may leave the body seriously depleted. An accident involving physical injury. A genetically prompted malfunction of an organ like the heart. A family death or major trauma. All these events can so undermine the immune systems of some young people that to rebuild health may be a long process.

From the first three months of life, when a breast-feeding mother sustains the immune potential of her child, to middle age and beyond, *prevention* of disease is far preferable to cure after the event. If the body does not succumb, there is a significantly reduced risk of viral damage to cells and the later disease or dysfunction that may result. Avoiding unnecessary disease is a positive way to sustain health in the long term. Prevention does not mean an obsessive avoidance of infection but the maintenance of conditions under which you are least likely to become sick. If situations present themselves that you know have the potential to be threatening, it is often possible to avoid that outcome.

For example, some people paint themselves into a corner in a legal dispute which sucks them inevitably into a traumatic and negative court battle. This not only undermines their economic resources because the costs are prohibitive, but it takes a heavy toll on their health. Would it not have been better to negotiate a settlement of the dispute, however disappointing, than to put one's health – even life – at risk? Another example is the pursuit of promotion and reward. Some people, offered an opportunity to progress which they cannot neglect, may impose great hardship and negative consequences on their families. Had they waited for another and less disruptive opportunity, everyone may have led a healthier life. Status and prosperity, as many people discover when they may have been irreparably harmed, are secondary to good health in later years.

A person with an efficient immune system will not become sick except under abnormal circumstances. Most of these fortunate people seldom or never get colds or other mild ailments though, because of genetic traits they have inherited, they may sometimes suffer from other chronic conditions unrelated to viral encounters.

This book came to be written for a surprisingly simple reason.

Most of my youth was spent near the sea, on the beach, and in the sun. Part of my working life took place in northern Europe and the rest in Australia. This meant there were times when I was deprived of adequate exposure to light and sunshine to which I had become accustomed. It was soon evident to me that there was a close correlation between sun and sickness.

My melanin levels had been activated in childhood and I was deeply suntanned. Whenever I maintained the suntan in the summer months, I remained free of illness in the winter. This became so obvious that I consciously set out to 'top up' my suntan in time for the European winter specifically to avoid illness. In part this was almost an obsession because, as a child in World War II, I had been seriously ill for a long period with TB and for many years after that I was unusually susceptible to upper respiratory infections. Sunlight solved this problem and today I only succumb to infection when sun deprived for a round of the seasons, or even longer.

On encountering the work of the immunologists and academics like Professor Lillyquist, it was obvious that their theories were not only rational but they had been adequately demonstrated in my life. I started to re-examine my own experience to analyse when and where any bouts of illness had occurred, and why. The correlation with sun exposure was undeniable.

However, in analysing why illness had occurred, it became obvious that the sunshine was only one element in a more complicated process of sustaining health. At this point it was necessary to delve deeper into medical research to identify all the elements that made avoidance of the common cold, and other ills, possible.

Let's attempt now to put these elements in some kind of perspective.

Physical fitness to a good general standard from childhood onwards is an essential basis for maximising immunity.

Childhood exposure to adequate light and sunlight is necessary to co-ordinate hormonal and metabolic systems and activate the skin protection provided by melanin (unless you're black skinned when the concern is to maintain adequate vitamin D levels).

Developing a positive approach to life and the ability to cope mentally and physically ensures that the work of the immune system is not compromised. Such attitudes are best developed in childhood following parental example. However, some young people may be motivated to counteract the unhealthy or negative attitudes of their parents and this reaction can also be a basis for good health.

Sustaining the physical resources of the body, and immunity, requires an adequate diet. Not a selection of foods based on fads or commercially promoted fashions but a good general diet that gives all the essential vitamins and minerals.

Maintaining adequate levels of vitamin A, C and E by the use of fresh fruit and other foods rich in these chemicals. Freshly squeezed orange juice is one way of providing these essentials.

Following the normal precepts of a long healthy life – sufficient rest and recreation, coping with the stresses of work and family life, acting positively to correct lifestyle anomalies and shortcomings, and avoiding excessive or debilitating demands on one's energy and emotional resources.

Getting enough time in the sun every day, preferably accompanied by fresh air and exercise.

At least once a year, but preferably throughout the summer months, if not spring and autumn, too, exposing your body to sunlight to the point where the melanin levels are activated strongly and you develop a healthy tan. If you happen to be fair skinned with blue eyes, it may still be possible to raise your melanin levels safely but this should be done gradually and with caution. Don't allow your skin to burn.

If you suffer a chronic condition for which you are taking medication on a long term basis, find out how the drug(s) may affect sun sensitivity or the function of the immune system. Some drugs, especially anti-inflammatory agents used to treat arthritis and high blood pressure or heart conditions, are known to inhibit immune response. Medical advisers who religiously follow the conventional view than the sun is an enemy may discourage the idea of exposing yourself to sunlight. The safest course is to experiment with care. You may well find you can reduce the medication, and that you will feel much healthier as a consequence. If you feel healthier, chances are you are.

Cigarette smoking appears to act adversely on the immune system so, if you have to smoke, stick to a pipe or cigars in moderation. A little of what you fancy, the saying goes, does you good...

Within a lifestyle that meets all or most of the basic health requirements, there are three specific anti-cold strategies that need to be restated:

1 Sunlight is the key. By programming your body and

manufacturing the essential hormone vitamin D from cholesterol circulating in the bloodstream, the sun not only keys up and maximises immunity but acts to prevent diseases, including internal cancers. The trick is to elevate melanin levels at a young age and maintain that protection for life. At all times avoid excessive exposure to the sun. People with activated melanin levels, however, often find they can remain in the sun for long periods without harm simply because their bodies are fully protected against UV radiation.

Ultimately, sun risk depends on skin type. The more pigment you carry, the darker your skin naturally and the darker your hair, the less likely you are to be adversely affected. If you are very blonde and apparently without pigment, brief sun exposures will be sufficient.

2 Ensure you receive sufficient anti-cold vitamins with a daily glass of fresh orange juice, the accent being on the word 'fresh'. The carton or bottled forms do not provide what you need. You have to start with a healthy looking real orange to work the trick. This, interacting with the effects of the sun and the production of vitamin D, is sufficient to maximise the protection needed by a healthy person.

3 Avoid the use of drugs – antipyretics like aspirin, antibacterial cough lozenges, cough remedies (except some of the suppressants), antibiotics unless essential to prevent a more serious outcome, and many so called 'cold cures' so you do not act against the good work of your immune system.

If you remain unconvinced that this strategy can rid you of colds, the regime is unlikely to work because your mind is saying to your immune system and the rest of your body that it isn't buying the deal.

Perhaps you are just sceptical.

If so, you can prove this approach by giving it a fair trial over a sufficient period of time (depending on your present lifestyle and immune resources). If your skin is lily white and as delicate as a soft leafed plant in the shadehouse, you can't suddenly start toasting yourself in the sun. You'll have to begin cautiously, say 10 minutes a day then increasing that time as you find you are 'hardening' off. You'll also shed some unwanted fat, too, and improve muscle tone significantly.

If, however, you're convinced – go for it. You have nothing to lose but your common cold.

In the early stages of changing the 'cold culture' and modifying your lifestyle to maximise immunity, you may have setbacks. Perhaps you will have been exposed to a virus that was simply unrecognisable by your immune system. Or you were, for whatever reason, 'run down' – perhaps after a long dark winter and sunlight deprivation. Perhaps you contracted another viral infection unrelated to the common cold which made heavy demands on your immunity and left you vulnerable. If this happens, there is a simple strategy for handling the unwanted symptoms that follow the initial immune response.

Pick the early indications that you are fighting off a cold virus – sore throat, the sniffles, swollen glands under the chin, feeling alternately hot and cold. Is this a coming cold, or a flu virus? You need to discriminate because the cold can be dealt with easily, the flu will have to run its natural course, preferably without the symptoms being suppressed to the point where the illness is prolonged (see pages 10-11).

If you are succumbing to a rhinovirus or coronavirus, or even a bacterially induced illness that is mimicking a common cold, you have a failsafe option until you can get your immunological act under way – let the symptoms indicating immune response take their course but head off the unwanted consequences.

You're streaming and this is both embarrassing and uncomfortable at work or in social encounters. If this process takes its course, you may well develop a cough when the excessive moisture drips constantly onto the lungs and, after a day or two, your nasal passages and airways will become congested with thick mucous. So don't let the streaming continue.

The moment the first signs are clearly established, boost your immunity in the ways outlined above, increase the intake of natural vitamins, and prevent streaming with a cold suppressant drug – but not one containing aspirin or paracetamol or any other antipyretic substance. If you do not allow the streaming to occur, you will not have to put up with the most objectionable manifestations of a cold, a stuffy nose and an inability to breathe normally.

The drug you are looking for contains atropine and/or in the case of cough suppressants, pseudoephedrine. Atropine and another chemical, hyoscine, are the main ingredients of belladonna, a medication that has been used for centuries. Atropine has a variety of uses but is essentially a 'drier'. Pseudoephedrine constricts blood vessels and helps to relieve the streaming from the nose and respiratory tract.

Atropine in a natural form is found in deadly nightshade, henbane and morning glory as well as other plants. The principal commercial source today is a shrub native to Australia, duboisia, once used by some Aborigines for medical and ceremonial purposes.

A word of caution.

Anyone on antihypertensives (drugs to control high blood pressure) or with enlargement of the prostate gland, should not use these preparations. Don't use them if you are abnormally thirsty or dehydrated – though it is unlikely you would be streaming in that case. And don't mix them with antidepressants, antihistamines or tranquillisers. Sufferers of glaucoma, Down's syndrome, or anyone with brain damage or dementia should avoid these products except under medical guidance. All this failsafe strategy does is prevent the unwanted outcome of the infection. It neither cures the cold nor aids the immune system in its task and should become unnecessary once you can get your immune system up to speed. But it means you can have a virtually 'coldless' cold and face the world in relative comfort even though it's a poor substitute for not getting the cold at all.

Suppressing the cold consequences will have to continue for up to 48 hours. Most of the tablets are effective for about 12 hours, so you may need to use four doses.

What do you do if you are taking antihypertensives? This is an interesting situation because the 'drying' effect of many of these medications may be sufficient to prevent streaming. Some, however, tend to dry the user for a period then, after he or she has been drinking to slake the resulting thirst, cause a sudden rehydration that can result in sneezing that looks, for half an hour or so, just like an oncoming cold.

Another word of caution.

Make sure that your diagnosis is correct. Often, particularly after a dry spell or period of drought, the onset of rains will cause sniffles and symptoms not unlike a coming cold but this is no more than the respiratory tract doing its usual job. A sniffle on its own may mean nothing until it is supported by some other clear sign or symptom that a virus is at work.

And a final caution.

The minefield of the mind can produce many curious physical responses. At one time it used to be considered wrong for people to be aware of symptoms because they could 'create' those symptoms, or mimic various diseases, if they were of a mind so to do. Medical practitioners deplored the medical encyclopedias that once sold in their millions for this reason. Self-diagnosis based on imperfect understanding and insufficient information can cause a lot of unnecessary anxiety in the fearful. Sometimes some people need to be sick for a host of perfectly rational psychological reasons. They can produce an illness almost to order to fulfil this objective even though there is no indication of actual disease – just inexplicable symptoms. Sometimes the immune system is tricked into presenting the signs and symptoms of disease, and immune response, when no viral agent is present – as appears to be the case with chronic fatigue syndrome. However, there's a lot to learn about that illness yet.

What is important here is not the negative capability of the mind, but the positive power it can unleash to prevent illness. If you really believe you are going to become ill, for whatever reason, you will succeed in hamstringing your immune system. If you are genuinely convinced that you'll remain well in the face of all viral, bacterial, fungal and other assaults, your immune system – if you've provided it with the necessary resources – can and will do the rest.

Conclusion

In this book we have assembled all the relevant information in the medical literature about the common cold. Going beyond that, a series of related studies have been introduced to show that the causes and origins of the cold are not as simple as pinning them down to a couple of hundred rhinoviruses, coronaviruses and types of flu. What we needed was an answer to a simple question: why do only some people fall ill when faced with these viruses while others remain healthy? And, more particularly, why do some people average three to six colds a year? The answers appear simpler than they are.

To develop a strategy for preventing colds we brought together some well tested ideas about the psychological areas of health working in concert with an efficient immune system. Why did some people's immune systems fail to intercept and destroy the ever present cold virus when it was activated under certain conditions?

In the Cleveland Family Study in the United States, the common cold - broadly defined to include related upper respiratory infections - accounted for 60 per cent of all sickness over a period of 10 years. That is a huge price to pay for loss of productivity, the plethora of largely useless medications, and in terms of inconvenience, discomfort and individual malaise. Nobel Prize winner Linus Pauling may have come up with the wrong answer in promoting massive doses of vitamin C but his theory at least focused attention on prevention and a possible explanation rooted in a form of deficiency.

When the concepts of sun and light deprivation were introduced, the whole mystery of cold susceptibility started to unravel. Like an Agatha Christie thriller, the guilty party was finally exposed - the sun. Or rather the cold sufferer who, denied adequate access to natural light and sunshine in industrial communities or in sun deficient environments, failed to compensate for needs established in the process of human evolution.

Let's draw these ideas together into a coherent explanation and strategy that summarises the view expressed in this book that construct the background of developing immunity.

Young children may inherit a degree of immunity to many viral and other assaults but their developing immune systems will have to 'see' many viruses and quickly create antibodies to promote effective resistance across a wide range of infections. If the conditions for maximising immunity are provided for the growing child, each infection that is seen and remembered by the immune system will not necessarily produce illness. However, it may produce signs that the immune system is functioning correctly to repel the invader. These signs should not be mistaken for 'illness' - they result in symptoms which need not be interfered with in normal circumstances except where a high fever threatens a very young child, or there is a risk of other complications. More of this in a moment.

As we looked at the Spitzbergen Study, it was tempting to accept the widely held idea that colds were the result of contact with infected individuals. This, however, was not born out in British research. It soon became obvious that no one could escape repeated contact with cold viruses, especially in winter months, yet only a quarter or fewer of these contacts resulted in an active infection.

We had to bracket out a separate condition, influenza, caused by one of only a few viruses which mutate genetically over time. A flu epidemic is usually the result of one 'new' form of the virus, though other forms are circulating at the same time and this can confuse diagnosis. Because the flu viruses are so few in number, and any one virus leading to a general outbreak of the illness can be identified from the previous 'season', a vaccine can be prepared and people most at risk can be protected. Not so with the cold because the potential sources of infection are so numerous.

Curious anomalies keep popping up.

Why, for example, are menstruating women so much more resistant to colds than at other times? This had to mean something. What happens in pregnancy that so boosts immunity? If only we could identify the factors responsible, we might be able to map out a course for cold prevention, more generally for reducing disease. Alongside this, it was important to tackle the antibiotic problem.

Antibiotics in the years following World War II, and even today, though less so, have been grossly over-prescribed and often wrongly prescribed. As a consequence, bacterial resistance to these wonder drugs began to build and their efficacy began to fall. Even worse, antibiotics are not even effective against a virus except in quite different circumstances and conditions.

Part of the problem here lay in the way we do medicine.

People were encouraged to involve their general practitioner in every cough and sniffle. The moment any symptoms developed, especially in children, the GP was called into the drama with the expectation that he would prescribe something. So he usually prescribed a high-tech antibiotic because lemon and honey seemed too simple, and going to bed with an aspirin hardly justified the consultation fee. No, his patients expected more than that. They expected to be cured. Most people never dreamt that the treatments most favoured - with the exception of going to bed with a lemon and honey drink - probably prolonged the illness, if it ever was an illness and not just normal immune function.

For years we had been busily removing tonsils, adenoids and many a grumbling appendix with nary a thought for the fact that they might have some value to their owners. One is reminded of 'doctor jokes' about getting children through private school on the proceeds of tonsillectomies. When it became known that these lymph glands were an essential part of the body's defences against disease, some physicians must have felt rather uncomfortable. Others just went on slicing out the offending organs when repeated tonsil infections struck their young patients. Fortunately, the human body is resilient and when you remove an organ like the spleen, for example, or even a kidney, a compensatory process occurs to make good the shortcoming.

Part of the problem we faced in proposing an end to the common cold lay in convincing you that processes like inflammation were a normal and healthy response, not a symptom of illness. A runny nose, nasal congestion, cough, headache and aching limbs were unwanted symptoms of illness - inflammation, tender glands, fever and fatigue were signs that everything was happening as it should. As a failsafe technique, we suggested that - if a cold virus gets through your defences and your immune system has to clobber it - steps to prevent the uncomfortable symptoms should make it possible for you to remain comfortable and presentable in public while resistance is built up to prevent another attack by that particular virus.

You may also have noticed that some viral infections go round the immunity 'ring' two or three times before you are finally immune, probably for life. We're not yet sure about this, however. Perhaps the immune system, under stressful circumstances, can 'forget' or fail to recognise an old adversary.

While recommending this intervention, it was necessary to stress that the wonder drug of past centuries, aspirin, was not the way to intercept or treat a cold. Sure it fixed the headache and dropped body temperature quickly, while ending some of the uncomfortable aches and pains that often accompany a high temperature. But it also inhibited the effective functioning of the immune system and reduced the immune resources of the body by affecting blood quality.

Aspirin is a great pain killer for people with conditions like arthritis. It has been heavily promoted in recent years as a NSAID, a means of reducing painful inflammation, a 'blood thinner' or anticlotting agent, and a constituent of various ointments to ease but not cure some skin conditions. But colds? No.

We moved to a position that saw succumbing to colds as a clear sign that something was amiss in the sufferer's immune system which, in some cases, could be sheeted back to diet, lifestyle, living and working environments, sunlight exposure and even mental attitude. There may be other as yet unidentified factors such as viral interference with one aspect of immune response. But given a change of lifestyle and attitude, supported by adequate dietary intake of the building blocks of immune resources, and the means of metabolising and synthesising these chemicals, it should be possible to correct this malfunction.

While it bore some resemblance to a British comedy film in the *Carry On* series, the Common Cold Research Unit in Britain provided research information on which to build an understanding of colds. Backed up by American and European research efforts, the nature and course of the common cold was thoroughly mapped. We soon learned that no one virus was responsible, cross-infection was largely a myth, and the chances of a cure were about nil.

By the time we got to the savage colds of the Scottish crofters, it was more than evident we were looking for something much more impressive than a tiny virus.

Working with these research results from so long ago, one feels a need for new studies of these relatively simple happenings, research conducted under the more stringent trial conditions imposed today. Many phenomena that seemed to be taken for granted 25 years ago cry out for detailed study and explanation. The feared crofters' cold was an example of a fascinating discovery. Why do, or did, crofters experience such serious viral infections? Is there something other than sunlight deficiency to explain this? I suspect there is.

Time and time again in digging up old research there seemed to be a much more rational interpretation than the conclusion reached at the time. With the benefit of hindsight, perhaps this was inevitable, but it left many important questions unanswered which, had they been resolved at the time, would have made it much easier to clarify the issues today. And to lay to rest finally the misleading statements still made regularly in today's media.

We took a detailed and rather technical look at the immune system and how it prevents illness in difficult circumstances, often despite the actions of the system's possessor. Were it not for the evolution of the immune system throughout human history and before, we would not exist as viable life forms. As a side issue, the vital importance of breast feeding as a part of the developing immune process became obvious. Some readers must have started to wonder whether we were paying a high price for the ignorance or prejudice of earlier times.

Implicit in much of this material was the role, or the dislocation, of the immune system in many other diseases, even autoimmune conditions like rheumatoid arthritis and AIDS.

Professor Dwyer's work on immunity and the NK cells, relative to stress and cancer susceptibility, ties in strongly with the beliefs of Professor Lillyquist. He holds that deep internal cancers may be prevented by sun exposure even though, for people with certain skin types, there is an increased risk of skin cancers. This is not new information. These facts have been known for 50 years at least.

That led to a confrontation of the concepts of 'mind' and 'body'.

Where do you draw the line. When does one process cease to be 'mind' and become 'body'? What, anyway, is the mind? Brain function? Some sensitive resonance of the whole organism? The coherent response of the senses mediated by intelligence? How can 'mind' impact on 'body' if they are both conceptual constructs invented simply to explain the difference between spontaneous physical action and discretionary conduct? Is the memory mind - or body? For our purposes, it would be easier to see mind and body as one.

Finally, we moved towards the idea that all these parts of the cold drama had to interact or interrelate to sustain health.

Without exposure to a strange virus, the immune system could not build resistance. Without physical exercise, metabolism was inhibited and slowed. A disturbed state of mind could undermine immune function. Without certain chemical resources and foods, the system would be deprived and eventually malfunction. If the co-ordinating effects of sun and light were denied, the processes of synthesis and co-ordination would be disrupted. All these interacting functions were essential to keep the body healthy. And each of us *relies* on the barriers put up by our immune system to outside attack.

At this point it became obvious that the three quarters of the population who do not succumb to a new virus, and whose immune systems have never 'seen' that antigen before so cannot recognise it until exposed, have an additional form of defence which may be inborn and, like melanin, has to be activated. We cannot identify this additional factor but we can maximise the good effects.

This comes down in the end to a very simple approach.

If you want to be rid of colds for life - given that the basic elements of good health are followed - consistent and safe exposure to sunlight for as much of the year as practically possible, coupled with the daily intake of natural vitamins from sources such as fresh squeezed orange juice, will maximise protection *if that is what you believe.*

Index

A
Acid medium 34
Acquired or specific immunity 9, 23, 52-53
ACTH 83
Adaptation 74, 82, 93
Adenoviruses 14, 18, 22, 31
Ageing 67, 73
Agricultural pest control 75
AIDS 54, 92, 118
Air conditioning 94, 102
Air hygiene 31
Air purifiers 31
Alcohol 48, 101
Alcoholism 81
Alternative or complementary practitioners 73
Amantadine 21-22
Analgesics 43
Andrewes, Sir Christopher 27-37, 75, 97
Anaemia 72
Animal breeding 75
Animal diseases 55
Animal fats 48-50
Anthrax 52, 54
Anthropological medicine 64
Anti-inflammatory agents 107
Antibiotics 7-8, 16, 40, 44-46, 55-56, 66, 71, 74, 83, 88, 99, 108, 115
Antibodies 11, 15, 19, 32-36, 44-46, 52, 56-57, 62, 66, 92, 103, 114
Antidepressants 83, 110
Antigen producing cells 52
Antigenic drift 19
Antigens 52-53, 56-57, 59, 66, 95-96, 103
Antihistamines 35, 110
Antiplatelet action 43
Antipyretics 63, 108, 109
Antiviral proteins 51
Appendix 52, 115
Arthralgia 21
Ascorbic acid 8, 69
Asian flu 20, 92
Aspirin 22, 40, 42-46, 62, 68, 108, 109, 115, 116
Asthma 17, 28, 43, 65
Athletes 41, 87
Atropine 110
Aurora 23

B
B-lymphocytes 52, 56
Bacteria 7-8, 13, 17, 21-25, 28, 31, 34, 44-45, 51-56, 61, 67, 78, 94-96, 108-109, 110, 115
Bassi, Augustino 54
Baume, Dr Peter 74
Bayer 43
Beliefs 61-63, 67-70, 91, 118
Belladonna 110
Bereavement 24, 87, 100
Beta-endorphins 68-69
Bikini Atoll 82
Bio-medicine 64
Blood circulation 68
Blood tests 73
Bone marrow 52, 56
Boston University School of Medicine 65, 91
Bowerchalke 33
Brain chemistry 61
Breast cancer 51
Breast feeding 9, 23, 104, 118
Bronchitis 13-14, 17, 18

C
Calcium 48-49, 79, 81
Calcium channel blockers 66

121

Cancer 24, 25, 31, 53, 54, 55, 57, 63, 67, 75, 79-82, 92, 108, 118
Cancer activating signal 57
Cancer research 63
Cancerous cells 57, 82
Candida albicans 56, 71
Capillary permeability 53
Carbohydrates 68
Carbon monoxide 94
Cardiovascular system 17
Cardiovascular disease 81
Central nervous system 17
Chemical messengers 63, 67-68
Chernobyl 25
Chicken pox 13
China 20
Chiropractors 73
Cholecalciferol 86
Cholesterol 48, 50, 77-78, 86, 108
Chronic fatigue syndrome 111
Chronic obstructive pulmonary disease 20
Cigarette smoking 50, 80, 92, 107
Circulatory system 72
Cleveland Family Study 14, 112
Coal miners 24, 58, 80, 86, 92
Coe virus 32
Cognitions 63
Cold culture 102, 108
Cold suppressants 40, 63
Cold transmission 8, 15-16, 32
Common Cold Research Unit 27, 35, 117
Community health 49
Commuting 96
Congestive heart failure 20, 44
Convulsions 99
Coping 63, 101, 104, 107
Cornell University 83-84
Coronaviruses 14, 16-18, 35, 109
Cortisol 67, 83
Coryza 18
Cough 15, 21-22, 30, 32-33, 45, 108, 109-110, 116

Cough lozenges 108
Coxsachie virus 14
Cross-infection 8, 29-34, 95, 117
Croup 17-18
Cyclo-oxygenase 68

D

Daily rhythms 86
Deadly nightshade 110
Defective genes 67
Dental caries 74, 81
Depression 81, 100
Dermatitis 79
Diabetes 81
Diagnosis 13, 21, 111, 114
Diesel fumes 94
Diet 8-9, 24, 40, 49-50, 57, 68, 70-74, 81, 87, 89, 106, 117
Digestion 68, 85
Dinorphins 69
Disinfectant sprays 31
DNA 54, 57
DNA repair 62
Dochez, Dr Alphonse 28
Dopamine 67
Down's syndrome 110
Drug misuse 7, 88
Drugs 10, 14, 19, 21-22, 41-45, 48, 50, 66-67, 77, 80, 83, 88, 96, 107-110, 115-116, 122
Duboisia 110
Dwyer, Professor John 54-57, 99-100, 118

E

E-coli 71
Echoviruses 14
Eilean nan Roan (Isle of Seals) 33
Electrical impulses 65
Electromagnetic fields 59, 94
Electromagnetic pulses 23
Electromagnetic spectrum 85
Electron microscopy 31
Emotional problems 94

Endocrine system 62, 85-86, 100
Endorphins 67-69
Enkephalins 67-69
Enteroviruses 18
Environmental adaptations 74
Environmental factors 34, 49, 93, 96
Enzymes 53, 68, 84
Ergocalciferol 86
Erythromycin 88
Ether 35
Evening primrose oil 73
Evolution 56, 74, 114, 118

F
Fatigue 16, 65, 83, 100, 111, 116
Fatty acids 51
Finsen, Niels 78
Fish oil 73, 81
Flu epidemics 19-23, 47, 96, 114-115
Flu injections 7, 47, 114-115
Flu viruses 14, 21, 35, 48, 96, 98, 109, 114-115
Fluorescent tubes 81-85, 92-93
Foetus 56
Folic acid 100
Food faddists 74
Food fibre 73
Foot and mouth disease 34-35, 54
Foreign proteins 53
Fructrose 58, 70
Full cream milk 49
Fungal agents 24
Funguses 53-54, 56, 92

G
Gallo, Dr Robert 54
Garlic 41, 61, 71-72
Gastric acidity 10, 40, 52
Gastrointestinal tract 51, 56
Genetics 7, 9, 19, 23, 53-55, 59, 62, 63-65, 67, 74-75, 78, 96, 104-105, 114
Glaucoma 117

H
Hahn, Robert A. 64
Hair loss 81
Harvard Hospital 28
Hay fever 30, 43
Hazardous cleaning agents 94
Headache 17, 21-22, 30, 43, 116
Healing resources 100
Health educators 80
Heliotherapy 79
Hemp 50
Henbane 110
Hepatitis 81
Hepatitis B carriers 92
Herbal remedies 73
Heroin 50
Herpes simplex 34
High blood pressure 43, 50, 66, 69, 75, 83, 88, 107, 110
High protein food 49, 68
High temperature 17, 43, 116
Hiroshima 64
Home medicines 45
Hormonal system 24, 48-49, 63, 67-68, 72-73, 81, 83, 85-86, 101, 103, 106, 108
Hufeland, Christopher 78
Human immunodeficiency virus (HIV) 54, 92
Hygiene 31, 41, 48
Hypertension 74
Hypothalamus 85-87
Hypothalamus-pituitary-adrenal axis 87

I
Immune enhancer 71
Immunoglobulin 101
Immunoregulation 66
Incubation periods 8, 16, 21, 31, 35-36
Infectious mononucleosis (glandular fever) 88
Inflammation 18, 43-44, 46, 53, 62, 68, 116

Influenza A 6, 14, 18-22, 35
Influenza B 6, 14, 18-22
Influenza C 14, 19
Innate immunity 52-53
Insecticides 94
Insomnia 81
Interferon 17-18, 22, 52
Iron deficiency 58, 72
Iron supplements 58
Irritability 81
Irritants 94

J
Jet travel 48
Jetlag 85
John Hopkins School of Hygiene 80
Junk foods 68, 96
Justice, Blair 61-68, 91

K
Kidneys 55
Killer cells 41
Kime, Dr Zane 76
Kindergarten 98
Kirby, Professor Janis 51
Koch, Robert 54

L
Laryngitis 14, 18
Lassitude 20
Legionnaire's disease 94
Lemon and honey 7, 12, 41-42, 45, 100, 102, 115
Lethargy 68
Leukaemia 25, 81
Liberman, Jacob 84-86
Lifestyle anomalies 107
Light intensity 27, 32, 86
Lillyquist, Professor M. J. 78-83, 106, 118
Liver 43-44, 54, 101
Loffler, Friedrich 54
Longevity 57, 89
Loss of appetite 30

Lung cancer 92
Lungs 94, 109
Lupus vulgaris 78
Lymph glands 52, 56-57, 115
Lymphocytes 52-53, 56, 66, 72, 99
Lymphoid organs 52

M
Macrophages 53
Magnesium 100
Magnetic storms 22
Malaise 21, 30, 113
Malaria 9, 53
Malnutrition 59
Maralinga 82
Margarine 48-49
Marijuana 50
Martinek and Berezin 85
Mass tourism 48
Measles 13, 48
Melanomas 23, 79-82
Melatonin 81, 83, 85-86
Menopause 48, 72
Menstrual cycle 16
Metabolic rate 42, 87, 100
Microwaves 59, 94
Mind/body hypothesis 9, 10, 24, 46, 60, 61-66, 73, 93, 101, 108, 111, 118
Morning Glory 110
Mucosal associated lymphoid tissue (MALT) 52
Mucous membrane 51, 101
Multicausal explanations 91
Multivitamins 61
Mumps 13
Muscle tone 78, 103, 109
Muscle wastage 87
Muscular aches 17
Myalgia 21

N
Narcotic drugs 69
Nasal symptoms 16, 21, 30, 109, 116

Nasal sprays 17
Natural opiates 69
Natural resistance 47
Naturopaths 73
Neuroactive chemicals 65
Neural connections 61
Neuroregulators 66
Neurotransmitters 63-69
Newcastle University 71
Niacin 100
Nicotine 50
NK cells 57, 118
Nosocomial infections 57
Novocain 69
NSAIDs 44, 116
Nuclear radiation 25, 52-53, 64, 82
Nutrition 41-42, 48-50, 58-59, 65, 70-71, 94

O

Oakley, Dr W. G. 28
Obesity 74, 87
Oestrogen 72
Oncogenes 57
Osteoporosis 48
Ott, Dr John 84
Over-training 87
Overcrowding 59

P

Pain killers 63, 67
Pandemics 20-21
Paracetamol 22, 42-46, 109
Parainfluenza virus 14, 18, 31
Parasites 54-55
Pasteur, Louis 54
Pathogens 9, 13-15, 23-25, 28, 43, 46-48, 51-54, 59, 65, 71, 91-95, 99, 102
Pathology 60
Pauling, Professor Linus 35-36, 69, 113
Peale, Norman Vincent 63
Peller, Dr Sigmund 80
Penicillin 55, 88

Peptide messengers 67
Peptides 69
Perfume additives 79
Peyer's patches 52
PH factor 51
Phagocytes 52
Pharyngitis 13, 18, 21
Photobiology 84
Photophobia 21
Photosensitivity 83
Photosynthesis 84-86
Physical fitness 103-104, 106
Physical stresses 93
Physical training 87, 103
Pigmentation 78, 82, 108
Pineal gland 85
Pipe and cigar smoking 50, 107
Placebos 28-29, 30, 36, 45
Plant propagation 75
Pneumonia 8, 13, 17, 20-23, 46, 55
Poisoning 45
Polio 13, 74
Polio epidemics 92
Pollutants 94, 96
Polyunsaturated margarine 49, 71
Poverty 59
Pre-eclampsia 43
Pregnancy 43, 56-57, 72, 115
Priest Island 32-33
Progesterone 72
Proprietary cold medicines 44
Prostaglandins 68
Prostate gland 110
Prostration 21, 30
Protozoa 54
Pseudo-healthy diets 58-59
Pseudoephedrine 110
Psycho-social factors 63
Psychology 60

R

Radiation 25, 64, 79, 82-83, 86, 108
Radio waves 23
Radioactive fallout 82

Radioactivity 64
Receptors 65-68, 100
Reed, Walter 54
Relaxation therapy 40
Reproduction 68, 72
Resistance resources 64, 91
Respiratory syncytial virus 14, 18
Rest 41-42, 100, 104, 107
Restricted spectrum lighting 59
Retina 79
Retrovirus 54, 92
Rheumatic fever 81
Rheumatoid arthritis 42, 118
Rhinitis 14
Rhinorrhea 16
Rhinoviruses 14, 16-18, 31, 34-36, 41, 88, 109, 112
Riboflavin 100
Rickets 49, 79
Rimantadine 22
RNA 54
Rommel, General 79-80
Rose, Robert 65

S

Salicylic acid 43
Salisbury, England 27-37
Saliva 16, 32
Salmonella 71
Salt intake 74
Schonlein, Johann 54
Self healing systems 63
Self-diagnosis 111
Sense of humour 61
Serotonin 68, 83
Serotypes 34
Serum cholesterol levels 50
Sex drive 81
Sexual maturation 83
Sexual potency 78, 80
Shift workers 93
Sick buildings 94
Sinusitis 13, 17, 30

Skin 21, 42, 51, 59, 77-84, 106, 107-108, 116, 118
Skin type 108, 118
Sleep deprivation 16
Slimming industry 87
Slow release patches 73
Smallpox 36, 74
Sneezing 16, 111
Solar flares 23
Solar therapy 79
Soluble mediators 53
Sore throat 16, 21, 31, 45-46, 88, 109
Spitzbergen Study 16, 32, 95, 114
Spleen 52, 116
St Bartholomew's Hospital 28
State of mind 24, 63, 66, 73, 118
Streptococci 11, 13-14, 17, 31, 40, 45, 65
Stress 24, 34, 36, 40-41, 47, 54, 57-58, 60, 63-66, 83, 88, 93-94, 97, 100-101, 104, 106, 116, 118
Stress hormones 83
Sucrose 70
Sun deprivation 86
Sun sensitivity 83, 107
Sunblock lotions 59
Sunburn 82
Sunglasses 59, 80, 83, 85
Sunlight cities 79
Sunspot activity 23, 96
Sunspot cycles 23
Suntan 79-83, 105
Sweet foods 68
Swollen glands 109
Sympathetic nervous system 85

T

T-cells 52, 56-57, 100
Tanning 78, 84
TB 30, 74, 78-79, 81, 92, 105
Tears 51
Testosterone 83
Tetracycline 83